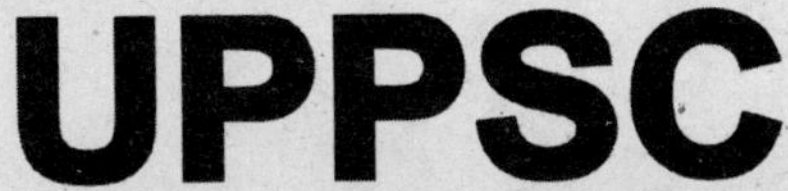

Uttar Pradesh Public Service Commission

MEDICAL OFFICER

Recruitment Examination

UPPSC

Uttar Pradesh Public Service Commission

MEDICAL OFFICER

Recruitment Examination

Part-I : General Knowledge

HOMEOPATHIC/AYURVEDIC

Dr. S.K. Bhatnagar

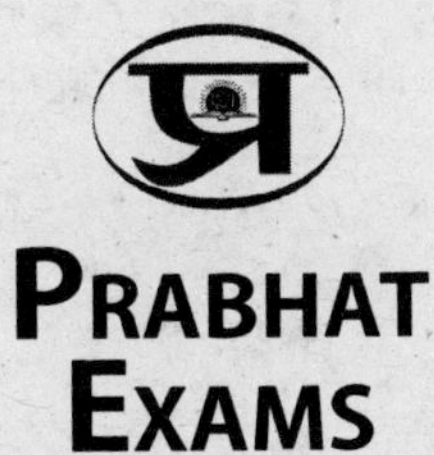

PRABHAT
EXAMS

Publisher

PRABHAT EXAMS

Imprint of Prabhat Prakashan Pvt. Ltd.

4/19 Asaf Ali Road, New Delhi–110 002

Ph. 23289555 • 23289666 • 23289777 • Helpline/ 7827007777

e-mail: prabhatbooks@gmail.com • Website: www.prabhatexam.com

Price

Two Hundred Ninety Five Rupees

ISBN 978-93-5322-054-9

Printed at

Maxcomm Prints, Delhi

UPPSC MEDICAL OFFICER
RECRUITMENT EXAMINATION
PART-1: GENERAL KNOWLEDGE
HOMEOPATHIC/AYURVEDIC
by Dr. S.K. Bhatnagar

ISBN 978-93-5322-054-9

₹ 295.00

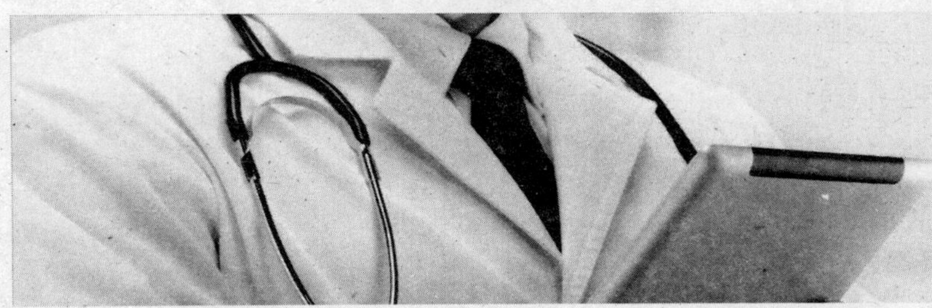

CONTENTS

General Knowledge

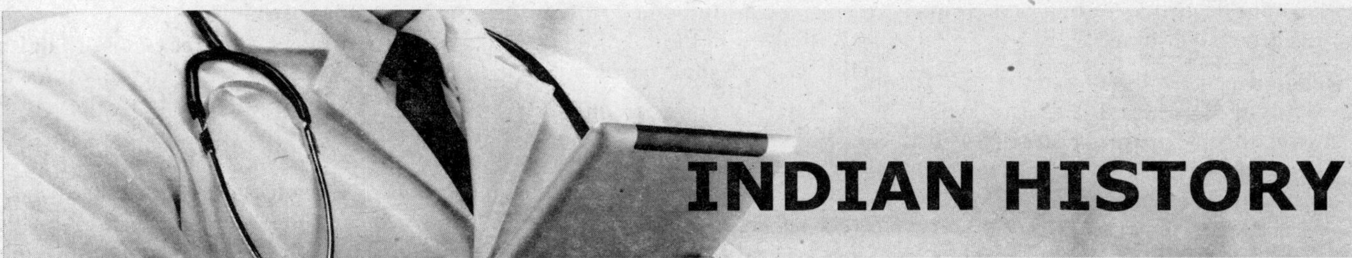

ANCIENT INDIA

Indus Valley Civilisation

- The most accepted period–2500 BC-1750 BC (by Carbon-14 dating).
- **John Marshall** was the first scholar to use the term 'Indus Valley Civilisation'.
- The Indus Valley Civilisation belongs to Proto-historic Period (Chalcolithic Age/Bronze Age).
- **Dayaram Sahni** first discovered Harappa Civilisation in 1921.
- **R.D. Banerjee** discovered Mohenjodaro or **Mound of the Dead** in 1922.

Vedic Culture (1500 BC-600 BC)

- Boghazkai inscription (Asia Minor, Turkey) proves Central Asian Theory as their homeland.
- The group that came to India first settled in the present Frontier Province and the Punjab–then called **Sapta Sindhu**, i.e. region of seven rivers.
- Vedic literature comprises four literary productions: (1) The Samhitas or Vedas; (2) The Brahmanas; (3) The Aranyakas; (4) The Upanishads.
- There are four Vedas–Rigveda, Samaveda, Yajurveda and Atharvaveda. The first three Vedas are jointly called Vedatrayi, i.e. trio of Vedas.

RigVeda

- The oldest religious text in the world.
- Collection of hymns, composed around 1700 BC, contains 1,028 hymns and is divided into 10 mandalas.
- The third mandala contains the **Gayatri Mantra**.

Samaveda (Book of Chants)

It is a collection of melodies. It contains Dhrupad Raga.

YajurVeda

The beliefs and rituals of non-Aryans are written in it.

AtharvaVeda

It is a book of **magical formula.**

The Upanishads

They define the doctrine of Karma, Atman (soul), Brahma (God), and origin of Universe. There are 108 Upanishads.

Vedangs

- They are the limbs of the Vedas. These are treaties of Science and Arts.
- **There are six Vedangs:**
  i. Shiksha (Phonetics)
  ii. Kalpa Sutras (Rituals)
  iii. Vyakarana (Grammar)
  iv. Nirukta (Etymology)
  v. Chhanda (Metrics)
  vi. Jyotisha (Astronomy)
- Panini wrote Ashtadhyayi (4th century BC) on Vyakarana.

Upavedas

There are four Upavedas:

- **Ayurveda** (Upaveda of the Atharvaveda)
- **Dhanurveda** (Upaveda of the Rigveda)
- **Gandharvaveda** (Upaveda of the Samaveda)
- **Sthapatyaveda** (Upaveda of the Yajurveda)

Puranas

There are 18 famous 'Puranas'. **Matsya Purana** is the oldest Puranic text.

Sutras

Sutra literature is divided into three classes:

i. Srauta Sutra–Dealing with large public sacrifices
ii. Griha Sutra–Dealing with rituals connected with birth, naming, marriage
iii. Dharma Sutra–Explain social and local customs

Smritis also known as

- **Dharma Shastra** are the law books.
- **Manav Dharma Shastra or Manusmirti** is the oldest and most famous.

Epic

There are mainly two **Mahakavyas** (Epics):

i. **The Ramayana (Valmiki):** It is known as **Adi Kavya** (the oldest epic of the world). At present, it consists of 24,000 shlokas.
ii. **The Mahabharata (Ved Vyasa):** The longest epic of the world. At present, it consists of 1,00,000 shlokas, i.e., verses in 18 Parvans, i.e., chapters, plus the Harivamsa supplement.

RigVedic/Early Vedic Period (1500–1000 BC)

Geographical Area

- Rigveda is the only source of knowledge for this period.
- Early Vedic people had knowledge of rivers Yamuna, Saraswati (Nandi tara) and Ganga, Ocean mentioned as Samudra (referred to collection of water and not sea), snow mountains (Himvat) and desert land (Dhawa).
- **The Purohita** or domestic priest was the first ranking official.
- Rigveda speaks of assemblies, such as the **Sabha, Samiti, Vidath and Gana**.
- Sabha was committee of few privileged and important individuals.

Society

- The Rig-vedic society comprised four varnas, namely **Brahmana, Kshatriya, Vaishya** and **Shudra**. This classification of society was based on the professions or occupations of the individuals.
- Child marriage was not in vogue.
- The cow was already deemed **Aghanya**, i.e. not to be killed.

- Alcoholic drinks, **Sura** and **Soma** were also consumed.

Religion

- **Indra, Agni** and **Varuna** were the most popular deities of Rigvedic Aryans. **Savitri was the god of light.** The famous Gayatri Mantra is addressed to her.
- Their religion primarily consisted of the worship of gods but **Yajna** or sacrifice became more important.

Later Vedic Period (1000 BC-600 BC)

With reference to the territorial divisions, the later Vedas give three broad divisions of India, viz. **Aryavarta** (Northern India), **Madhyadesa** (Central India) and **Dakshinapath** (Southern India).

Magadha Empire

- The period from 6th century BC to 4th century BC saw the struggle for supremacy among four mahajanapadas–Magadha, Kosala, Vatsa and Avanti.
- The founder of Magadha was **Jarasandha** and **Brihadratha**.

Nanda Dynasty (344 BC-323 BC)

Mahapadmananda

- The Shishunaga dynasty was overthrown by **Mahapadma**.
- It is considered to be the first non-Kshatriya dynasty and ruled for 100 years.
- He conquered **Kosala** and **Kalinga**.

Dhanananda

- The last king Dhanananda is possibly identical with the **Agrammes** or **Xandrames** of the Greek texts.
- It was during the rule of Dhanananda that the invasion of Alexander took place in north-west India in 326 BC.
- The Nanda dynasty came to an end about 322–21 BC and was supplanted by another dynasty known as Mauryas, with **Chandragupta Maurya** as the founder.

Religious Movements (600 BC-400 BC)

Buddhism: Buddha's Life

Gautama Buddha, founder of Buddhism, was born in 563 BC (widely accepted), on the Vaishakha Purnima day at **Lumbinivana** in **Kapilvastu** (now situated in the foothills of Nepal) in the **Sakya Kshatriya** clan.

Major Events of Buddha's Life

Events	Symbols
Janma (Birth)	Lotus and Bull
Mahabhinishkramana (Renunciation)	Horse
Nirvana (Sambodhi Enlightenment)	Bodhi tree
Dharmachakra Paravartan First Sermon	Wheel
Mahaparinirvana (Death)	Stupa

Teachings of Buddha

(a) His four Noble Truths:

1. The world is full of sorrows.
2. The cause of sorrow is desire, Dwadash Nidan/Pratitya Samutpada.
3. If desires are conquered, all sorrows can be removed, Nirvana.
4. This can be achieved by following the eight-fold path, Ashtangika Marga.

(b) Eight-fold Path:

(Ashtangika marga)

- Right understanding
- Right thought
- Right speech
- Right action
- Right livelihood
- Right effort
- Right mindfulness
- Right concentration.

(c) Three Jewels (Triratnas):

- Buddha
- Dhamma
- Sangha

Buddhist Sangha

It consisted of monks (Bhikshus or Shramanas) and nuns, who acted as a torchbearer of the dhamma. The worshippers were called upasakas.

Jainism

- It was founded by Rishabhnath.
- According to Jain tradition, there were 24 **Tirthankaras** the first being Rishabhadeva/Adinatha and the last being Mahavira.
- The name of two Jain Tirthankaras–**Rishabha** and **Arishtanemi** are found in the **Rigveda**.

Doctrines of Jainism

- **Triratnas, i.e., Three Gems of Jainism**
  1. **Samyak Shradha/Vishwas (right faith):** It is the belief in Tirthankaras.
  2. **Samyak Gyan (right knowledge):** It is the knowledge of the Jain creed.
  3. **Samyak Karma/Acharana (right action/conduct):** It is the practice of the five vows of **Jainism**.

Five Carinal Principles

- Non-injury (Ahimsa).
- Non-lying (Satya).
- Non-stealing (Asteya).
- Non-possession (Aparigraha).
- Observing continence (Brahmacharya).

- The first four principles were given by Parshvnath while fifth was added by Lord Mahavira.

Jain Literature

- The sacred literature of the Svetambaras is written in a **Prakrit**.
- The important Jain texts are: (i) **Kalpasutra** (in Sanskrit)–Bhadrabahu, (ii) **Bhadrabahu Charita**, (iii) **Parishishta Parvan** (an appendix of **Trishashthi-shalaka Purush**) –Hemchandra.

Jain Councils

- First Jain council was held at Pataliputra in the fourth century BC under the leadership of Stulabahu.
- Second Jain council was at Vallabhi in Gujarat in third century under the leadership of Aryaskandil Nagarjuna Suri.
- Third Jain council was held at Vallabhi in 5th century A.D. under the leadership of Devardhi Kshama Sramana.

Origin of the Mauryas

Chandragupta Maurya (322 BC-298 BC)

- Also called **Sandrocottus/Androcottus** by the Greek scholars.
- He dethroned the last Nanda ruler Dhanananda and founded the Mauryan dynasty with capital at Patliputra.
- Chandragupta defeated Seleucus I Nicator, the general of Alexander in North-West India in 305 BC.
- Seleucus sent a Greek Ambassador, **Megasthenes**, to the court of Chandragupta Maurya.

- Chandragupta embraced Jainism and went to Chandragiri Hill, at Shravanbelagola with Bhadrabahu, where he died of slow starvation (Salekhan).
- Chandragupta was the first Indian ruler to unite the whole North India.

Ashoka (273 BC-232 BC)

- He was the greatest Mauryan ruler whose empire extended to the whole of sub-continent except extreme south. It included Afghanistan, Baluchistan, Kashmir and valleys of Nepal.
- According to Buddhist tradition, Ashoka usurped the throne after killing his 99 brothers and spared **Tissa**, the youngest one.
- Ashoka had himself formally crowned in 269 BC.
- Ashoka fought the **Kalinga War** in 261 BC in the 9th year of his coronation.
- He embraced Buddhism under **Upagupta**.
- He sent his son Mahendra and daughter Sanghamitra to Ceylon as Buddhist missionaries with a sapling of original peepal tree.
- He inaugurated **Dhamma Yatras** from the 11th year of his reign by visiting Bodh Gaya; also appointed Dhamma Mahamatras (officer of righteousness to spread the message of Dhamma).

Ashoka's Dhamma

Its broad objective was to preserve the social order it ordained that people should obey their parents, pay respect to Brahmans and Buddhist monks show mercy to slaves and servants.

Later Mauryas (232 BC-185BC)

The last Mauryan ruler, **Brihadratha**, was assassinated in 185 BC by his commander-in-chief, **Pushyamitra Sunga**.

Post-Maurya/Pre-Gupta Period (185 BC-319 AD)

The Sunga Dynasty (185 BC to 73 BC)

- Sunga Dynasty was established by **Pushyamitra Sunga**, a Brahmin Commander-in-Chief of the last Mauryan ruler named Brihadratha in 185 BC.
- He is considered to be the persecutor of Buddhism.
- Pushyamitra was succeeded by his son **Agnimitra**, the hero of Kalidasa's drama **Malavikagnimitra**.
- **Patanjali**, author of the **Mahabhasya** was the priest of two Ashvamedha Yaggas, performed by Pushyamitra Sunga.
- The famous book on Hindu law **Manusmriti** was compiled during this period.

Kanva Dynasty (73 BC-28 BC)

- In 73 BC, Devabhuti, the last ruler of the Sunga dynasty, was murdered by his minister **Vasudeva**, who usurped the throne and founded the Kanva dynasty.
- The last ruler, Susarman, was killed by Andhra King, Simuka.

Satavahana Dynasty (60 BC-225 AD)

Capital–Pratishthan-Paithan (Maharashtra)

- **Simuka** (60 BC-37 BC) was the founder of the Satavahana Dynasty.
- **Gautamiputra Satakarni** revived the Satavahana power and defeated the Saka Ksatrap Snehapana. He was the greatest Satavahana ruler.
- **Pulamayi III** was the last Satavahana ruler.
- **Stupas:** The most famous of these attributed to the Satavahana period are **Amravati**, a sculptural treasure house, and **Nagarjunakonda**.
- The official language of the Satvahanas was **Prakrit**.

Foreign Successors of Mauryas

The Sakas (1st Century BC-4th Century AD)

- The **Sakas**, also known as **Scythians**, replaced the Indo-Greeks in India.
- The most famous Saka ruler in India was **Rudradaman** (130 AD).
- In about 58 BC, the king of Ujjain, Vikramaditya is supposed to have fought effectively against the Sakas. An era called **Vikrama Samvat** is reckoned from 58 BC.

The Kushanas (1st Century AD-3rd Century AD)

- Kushanas replaced the Greeks and Parthians.
- Their capitals were at **Peshawar (Purushapura)** and **Mathura**.
- The most famous Kushana ruler was Kanishka, also known as 'Second Ashoka'. He started an era in 78 AD which is now known as the **Saka Era** and is used by the Government of India.
- Kanishka was a great patron of Mahayana Buddhism. In his reign, **4th Buddhist Council** was held in **Kundalavana**, **Kashmir** where the doctrines of the Mahayana form of Buddhism were finalised.
- The Kushanas controlled the famous **silk route**.
- The Kushanas were the first rulers in India to issue gold coins on a wide scale.
- In the royal court of Kanishka, a host of scholars found patronage. **Parsva, Vasumitra, Asvaghosha, Nagarjuna, Charaka** and **Mathara** were some of them.
- Kushana Empire gave rise to Gandhara and Mathura Schools of Art.
- Vatsyayana wrote **Kamasutra** in this period.

Gupta Period (319 AD-540 AD)

- This period is referred to as the Classical Age or Golden Age of ancient India.
- Sri Gupta was the founder of the Gupta dynasty. Sri Gupta was followed by his son Ghatotkacha and he was followed by his son Chandragupta. Both used the simple title of Maharaja.

Chandragupta I (319AD-334 AD)

- He was the first Gupta ruler to assume the title of **Maharajadhiraja**.
- He started the **Gupta Era** in 319AD-320 AD.

Samudragupta (335AD-380 AD)

- Samudragupta was the greatest king of the Gupta dynasty.
- Samudragupta's military campaigns justify description of him as the **Napoleon of India** by **V.A. Smith**.

Chandragupta (II) (380AD-414 AD)

- **Chandragupta II conquered Western Malwa and Gujarat, from the Shaka Kshatrapas Rudrasena III.**
- He issued silver coins in the memory of victory over Sakas. He was the first Gupta ruler to issue silver coins and adopted the titles **Sakari** and **Vikramaditya**.

- It was in Chandragupta's time that the Chinese pilgrim **Fahien** visited India.

Navratna (Nine Gems) of Chandragupta II

1. Kalidasa (Poetry: Ritusamhara, Meghadutam Abhijnan Shakuntalam).
2. Amarsinh (Amarsinh Kosha)
3. Dhanvantri (Navanitakam medicine text)
4. Varahamihira (Pancha Siddhantika)
5. Vararuchi
6. Ghatakarna
7. Kahapranak
8. Velabhatta
9. Shanku

Kumaragupta I (415AD-455AD)

He founded the **Nalanda Mahavihara** which developed into a great centre of learning.

Skandagupta (455AD-467 AD)

- He repulsed the ferocious Hunas' attacks twice. The heroic feat entitled him the title **Vikramaditya** (Bhitari Pillar Inscription).
- During his period, Sudarshana Lake was repaired and its embankments were rebuilt.

Contribution of Gupta Rulers

- **City Administration:** Paura was the council responsible for city administration.
- **Army Military:** Chariots receded into the background and **cavalry** came to the forefront.
- **Senabhakta:** It was a form of tax.
- **Revenue:** Land revenue was the chief source of states' income.
- **Judiciary:** For the first time, civil and criminal laws were clearly defined and demarcated.
- **Coinage:** Guptas issued the largest number of gold coins, which were called **Dinaras** in their inscriptions. Silver coins were called **Rupayakas**.

MEDIEVAL INDIA

Delhi Sultanate (1206 AD-1526 AD)

- First Muslim invasion by Mohammad bin Qasim (712 AD).
- First Turkish Invasion by Mahmud Ghaznavi (998 AD-1030 AD): Sultan Mahmud of Ghazni. In 1025, he attacked and raided the most celebrated Hindu temple of Somnath.

Mahmud of Ghazni

- He patronised three persons, contemporary to him: **Firdausi** (court poet), **Al Beruni** (scholar) and **Utbi** (court historian).
- Al Beruni wrote Kitab-ul-Hind.
- Mahmud is said to have made **17 raids** into India. A decisive battle between Mahmud and Anandpala was fought in 1008AD-1009 AD at **Waihind** during his sixth expedition.
- In 1194 AD, Jaichand of Kannauj was also defeated at the **Battle of Chandawar**.
- **Second Turk Invasion-Mohammad Ghori's invasion (1175 AD-1206 AD):** Mohammad Ghori invaded India and laid the foundation of the Muslim domination in India. He may be considered the founder of Muslim rule in India.

The Slave Dynasty (1206 AD-1290 AD)

Qutubuddin Aibak (1206 AD-1210 AD)

- A Turkish slave by origin after the death of Ghori, Aibak founded the Slave Dynasty in 1206 AD. For his generosity, he was given the title of **Lakh Baksh** (giver of lakhs).
- He died in 1210 AD while playing **Chaugan** or polo.
- He constructed two mosques, **Quwwat-ul-Islam** in Delhi and **Adhai din ka Jhonpra** in Ajmer. He also began the construction of **Qutub Minar**, in honour of famous Sufi Saint, **Khwaja Qutubuddin Bakhtiyar Kaki**.

Aram Shah (1210 AD)

After Qutubuddin's death, his son Aram Shah succeeded him.

Razia Sultan (1236 AD-1240 AD)

She was the first and Muslim woman ruler of Medieval India.

Balban (1266 AD-1287 AD)

- He himself was a member of Chalisa or Chahalgani but he broke the power of Chahalgani and restored the prestige of the crown.
- He created a strong centralised army and established the military department **Diwan-i-Arz**. He ordered the separation of military affairs from finance department (Diwan-i-Wazarat).

The Khilji Dynasty (1290 AD-1320 AD)

Jalaluddin Khilji

- He was the first ruler of Delhi Sultanate to clearly put forward the view that the state should be based on the willing support of the governed and that since the large majority of the people in India were Hindus, the state in India could not be a truly Islamic State.
- The most important aspect of his reign was invasion of Devagiri in 1294 AD by his nephew and son-in-law Alauddin Khilji.

Alauddin Khilji (1296 AD-1316AD)

- He came to the throne by treacherously murdering his uncle and father-in-law Jalaluddin Khilji.
- He was the first Turkish Sultan who separated religion from politics.

The Tughlaq Dynasty (1320 AD-1414 AD)

Ghiyasuddin Tughlaq

- Ghazi Malik or Ghiyasuddin Tughlaq was the founder of Tughlaq dynasty.
- He was the first sultan of Delhi who took up the title of Ghazi or **slayer of the infidels**.
- **Construction of canals** and formulation of a **famine policy**.
- Started the barter system or sharing of crops.
- He built the city of **Tughlaqabad** near Delhi and made it his capital.
- Sufi saint, Shaikh Nizam-ud-din Aulia said Delhi is far away in regard to him.
- He died in 1325 AD, after a fall from a high-raised pavilion.

Mohammad Bin Tughlaq (1325AD-1351AD)

- Prince **Jauan**, son of Ghiyasuddin Tughlaq, ascended the throne in 1325 AD.

- Transfered the Capital (1327 AD) from Delhi to Devagiri, which was thus named Daulatabad.
- The famous Moroccan traveller Ibn Batuta came to Delhi in 1334 AD and acted as the Qazi of the capital for eight years. He recorded the contemporary Indian science in his **Safranamah** (Rahela).

Firoz Shah Tughlaq (1351 AD-1388 AD)

- He decreed that whenever a noble died, his son should be allowed to succeed to his position.
- It was during the time of Firoz that **Jizya** became a separate tax. Firoz refused to exempt the Brahmanas from payment of Jizya.
- He was a great builder. The cities of Fatehabad, Hisar, Jaunpur and Firozabad stand to his credit.
- Barani, the historian, was in his court. He wrote **Tarikh-i-Feroshahi** and **Fatwa-i-Jahangiri**.

Timur's Invasion (1398 AD-1399 AD)
Timur, the lame, a Turkish Chief invaded India in 1398 during the reign of **Muhammad Shah Tughlaq**, the last ruler of Tughlaq dynasty. Timur returned to Central Asia, leaving a nominee named Khizr Khan to rule in Punjab.

The Lodhi Dynasty (1451 AD-1526 AD)

Bahlol Lodhi (1451 AD-1488 AD)

- Founder of Lodhi dynasty in India.
- Never sat on throne, used to sit on carpets along with Anines.

Sikandar Lodhi (1489 AD-1517 AD)

- Noblest of the three Lodhi rulers, real name was **Nizam Khan** (son of Bahlol Lodhi).
- He built a new city named Agra, and made it his capital.
- He was a poet and wrote verses in Persian under the pet name **Gularukh**.

Ibrahim Lodhi (1517 AD-1526 AD)

- He was the last king of the Lodhi dynasty and the last sultan of Delhi.
- He was defeated and killed at the hands of Babur in the **First Battle of Panipat in 1526 AD**.

Amir Khusro

- He was a Persian poet (1253 AD-1325 AD) associated with royal courts of more than seven rulers of the Delhi Sultanate.
- He was also a musician, he invented sitar.
- He innovated **Khayal** (a style of singing).
- In his book **Tarikh-i-Alai**, he gave an account of conquest of Alauddin Khilji.
- He also lived in the court of Ghiyasuddin Tughlaq and wrote **Tughlaqnamah**.
- Khusro is also known as **Tuti-i-Hind** or 'Parrot of India'.

Vijayanagar and Other Kingdoms

Vijayanagar Empire (1336 AD-1580 AD)

- Vijayanagar kingdom and the city were founded by Harihar and Bukka.
- They were brought to the centre by Muhammad-bin-Tughlaq, converted to Islam and were sent to South to control rebellion but motivated by a Bhakti saint Vidyaranya, they established Vijayanagar kingdom in 1336 AD.
- Vijayanagar period can be divided into four distinct dynasties, viz. Sangam, Saluva, Tuluva and Aravidu.

Bahamani Kingdom

- The Bahamani kingdom of Deccan was founded by **Hasan Gangu**. The capital was Gulbarga. Hasan Gangu took the title of Alauddin Hasan Bahaman Shah and became the first king of Bahaman in 1347 AD.
- The last ruler of Bahamani kingdom was **Kalim Ullah Shah**.
- **Nizam Shahis of Ahmadnagar**. Founder–Ahmad Nizam Shah, later annexed by Shahjahan.
- **Muhammad Quli Qutab Shah** was the greatest of all. He founded the city of **Hyderabad**. He built the famous **Charminar**. The kingdom was annexed by Aurangzeb (1687 AD).

Mughal Period (1526 AD-1540 AD and 1555 AD-1857 AD)

Babur (1526 AD-1530 AD)

- The foundation of the Mughal rule in India was laid by Babur in 1526 AD.
- Babur defeated **Ibrahim Lodhi** in the **First Battle of Panipat** on April 21, 1526 AD and established the Mughal dynasty.
- In 1527 AD, he defeated **Rana Sanga** of Mewar at **Khanwa**.
- In 1528 AD, he defeated **Medini Rai** of **Chaneri** at **Chanderi**.
- In 1529 AD, he defeated Muhammad Lodhi (uncle of Ibrahim Lodhi) at **Ghaghra**.
- He wrote his autobiography **Tuzuk-i-Baburi** in Turki language.

Humayun (1530 AD-1540 AD and 1555 AD-1556 AD)

- His first campaign was against **Kalinjar**.
- **Battle of Chausa** (1539 AD) was fought between **Sher Shah** and **Humayun's** army. **Humayun** was badly defeated and escaped. He was saved by **Nizam**.
- **Battle of Kannauj (Bilgrama) (1540 AD):** Humayun was again defeated by Sher Shah.
- **Bairam Khan**, his most faithful officer, helped him. After the battle of Machhiwara against the Afghans and battle of Sirhind against Sikandar Shah, Humayun's second coronation was organised.
- His sister, **Gulbadan Begum** wrote his biography **Humayunama.**

Sher Shah Suri and the Afghan Empire (1540 AD-1555 AD)

- His real name was **Farid**.
- He usurped the throne as 'Hazarat-i-Ala'.
- **Battle of Chausa:** In 1539 AD, he captured Chausa from Humayun. He assumed the title of Sher Shah as the emperor.
- **Malik-Mohammed Jayasi** wrote **Padmavat** (Hindi) during his reign.

Akbar (1556 AD-1605 AD)

- Akbar, the eldest son of Humayun, ascended the throne under the title of **Jalaluddin Muhammad Akbar Badshah Ghazi** at the young age of 14 at **Kalanaur, Punjab** and his tutor **Bairam Khan** was appointed as the regent.
- **Second Battle of Panipat (5th November, 1556)** was fought between **Hemu** (the Hindu General of Muhammad Adil Shah) and **Bairam Khan** (the regent of Akbar). **Hemu** was defeated, captured and slained by **Bairam Khan**.

- He also ended the interference from **Peticoat Government** (1560 AD-1562 AD) represented by **Maham Anaga** and **Adham Khan Junta**.
- The **Battle of Haldighati** (1576 AD) was fought between **Rana Pratap** of Mewar and Mughal army led by **Man Singh** of Amer. Rana Pratap was defeated.
- Akbar proclaimed a new religion, Din-i-Ilahi, in 1581 AD.
- Birbal was the only Hindu who followed this new religion Din-i-Ilahi. However, it did not become popular.
- Tulsidas **(Ramcharitmanas)** also lived during Akbar's period.
- Abul Fazal wrote ***Akbarnama***, the appendix of which was called **Ain-i-Akbari**.

Navratnas in Akbar's Court

1. **Abul Fazal**
2. **Faizi**
3. **Tansen**
4. **Birbal**
5. **Raja Todar Mal**
6. **Raja Man Singh I**
7. **Abdul Rahim Khan-I-Khana**
8. **Fakir Aziao-Din**
9. **Mulla Do-Piyaza**

Jahangir (1605 AD-1627 AD)

- Salim, son of Akbar, came to the throne after Akbar's death in 1605 AD.
- In 1608 AD, **Captain William Hawkins**, a representative of East India Company, came to Jahangir's court. **Sir Thomas Roe**, an ambassador of King James I of England, also came to his court. Jahangir granted permission to the English to establish a trading port at Surat.
- He wrote his memories **Tuzuk-i-Jahangiri** in Persian.

Shahjahan (1628 AD-1658 AD)

- His real name was **Khurram**. He was the youngest prince to be appointed as governor of Deccan at the age of 15.
- His beloved wife **Mumtaj Mahal** (original name **Arzumand Bano**) died in 1631 AD. To perpetuate her memory, he built the Taj Mahal at Agra in 1632 AD-1653 AD.
- The **Red Fort**, **Jama Masjid** and **Taj Mahal** are some of the magnificent structures built during his reign.
- Shahjahan was imprisoned by his son Aurangzeb in the Agra Fort, where he died in captivity in 1666 AD. He was buried in the Taj (Agra).

Aurangzeb (1658 AD-1707 AD)

- After the victory of Samugath, Aurangzeb was crowned at Delhi under the title Alamgir.
- Aurangzeb compiled **Fatwa-i-Alamgiri**.
- He was called **Zinda Pir**, the living saint.
- **Jat** revolted under **Gokla Rajaram and Churaman**.

Marathas

Shivaji (1627 AD – 1680 AD)

- He had established an independent Maratha Kingdom.
- In 1674, he was formally crowned as the Chhatrapati
- He promoted the usage of Marathi and Sanskrit.

Sambhaji (1680 AD-1689 AD)

He provided protection and support to **Akbar II**, the rebellious son of Aurangzeb.

Rajaram (1689 AD-1700 AD)

Rajaram created the new post of **Pratinidhi**, thus taking the total number of ministers to nine (Pratinidhi + Ashtapradhan).

The Peshwas (1713 AD-1880 AD)

Balaji Vishwanath (1713 AD-1720 AD)

- Shahu honoured him with title of 'Sena Karta' in 1708 AD and made him his Peshwa in 1713 AD.
- He concluded an agreement with the Sayyed brothers, by which the Mughal emperor, Farrukhsiyar recognised Shahu as the King of Swarajya.

Baji Rao (1720 AD-1740 AD)

- Maratha power reached its zenith under him.
- He conquered Salsette and Bassein in 1733 AD. He also defeated the Nizam-ul-Mulk near Bhopal and concluded the treaty of **Durai Sarai**, by which he got Malwa and Bundelkhand (1737 AD).

Balaji Baji Rao Nana Sahib (1740 AD-1761 AD)

In the third Battle of Panipat in 1761 AD between the Marathas and Ahmad Shah Abdali, Viswas Rao, the son of Nana Sahib, died.

The Advent of Europeans

Portuguese

- The Cape route was discovered from Europe to India by **Vasco da Gama**.
- He reached the port of Calicut on May 17, 1498 AD and was received by the Hindu ruler of Calicut (known by the title of **Zamorin**).
- The first Governor of Portuguese in India was Francisco Almeida (1509 AD). He introduced "The Policy of Blue Water".
- First Portuguese factory was established at Calicut.

Dutch

- The Dutch East India Company established factories in India at Masulipatnam in 1605 AD, Pulicat (1610 AD), Surat (1616 AD), Bimlipatam (1641 AD), Karaikal (1645 AD), Chinsura, Kasimbazar, Patna, Balasore, Nagapatam and Cochin.
- The Dutch conceded to British after their defeat in the Battle of Sedera in 1759 AD.

English

The Governor and company of merchants of London trading into the East Indies, popularly known as the English East India Company, were formed in 1600 AD.

British East India Company

- The first factory was built in Surat (1608 AD). Surat was replaced by Bombay and made the headquarters on the West coast in 1687 AD.
- In 1717 AD, John Surman obtained royal farman from the Mughal emperor Farrukhsiyar. This farman is also called the Magna Carta of the British rule in India as it gave large concessions to the company.

MODERN INDIA

Expansion of British Power

Bengal

- **Battle of Plassey:** On 23rd June, 1757 AD, English won the battle against Siraj-ud-Daula, and compelled the Nawab to concede all the demands.
- **Battle of Buxar:** Mir Qusim formed an alliance with Nawab of Awadh, Shuja-ud-Daula, and Mughal Emperor Shah Alam-II and fought with the British army at Buxar on 22nd October, 1764 AD.

Impact of Victory of Plassey and Buxar

- Victory of Plassey laid the foundation of British rule in India and made them a powerful factor in Bengal politics.
- Victory of Buxar established English supremacy over whole of North India as the emperor of Hindustan was defeated.

Treaty of Allahabad (August 1765 AD)

English got the Diwani right (right to collect revenue) of Bengal, Bihar and Orissa and gave Rupees 26 lakh.

Drain of Wealth

'Drain of Wealth' theory refers to an importation of national product of India, which was not available for consumption to its people.

Indian Renaissance

Arya Samaj

- The first Arya Samaj unit was founded by Swami Dayanand Saraswati in 1875 AD in Bombay.
- He looked on the Vedas as 'India's Rock and Ages'. His mottos were **Go back to Vedas** and **India for the Indians**.

Ramakrishna Mission

It was established by Swami Vivekananda to carry on relief and social work after death of his **Guru Rama Krishna Paramahansa** in 1897 AD.

Swami Vivekananda

- His original name was **Narendranath Dutt**.
- He attended the Parliament of Religions held at Chicago in 1893 AD and published two papers, **Prabhudhha Bharat** in English and **Udbodhana** in Bengali.
- He was considered as the spiritual father of the modern nationalist movement.

Veda Samaj

It is called Brahmo Samaj of South. It was started by Sridharalu Naidu.

The Prarthana Sabha

- It was founded in 1867 AD by M.G. Ranade.
- Prominent leaders were Dr. Atmaram Pandurang and R.G. Bhandarkar and N.G. Chandavarkar.

Young Bengal Movement

- It was founded by **Henry Louis** and **Vivian Derozio**.
- They believed in truth, freedom and religion. It supported women's education.

Indian Reform Association

It was founded by **Keshab Chandra Sen** in Calcutta in 1870 AD.

Theosophical Society

The Theosophical Society India was founded by **Annie Besant**. She founded Central Hindu College in 1898 AD, which became Banaras Hindu University in 1916 AD.

Deccan Education Society

- Founded by **M.G. Ranade, V.G. Chibdonkar** and **G.G. Agarkar** in Pune in 1884 AD.
- The society founded the **Ferguson College**.

The Servants of India Society

Founded by **Gopal Krishna Gokhale** in Bombay in 1905 AD.

Poona Seva Sadan

Founded by G.K. Devdhar and Ramabai Pande in Pune.

Nishkam Karma Math

- Founded by **Dhondo Keshav Karve** in Pune.
- Founded India's first Women's University in Pune in 1916.

The Bharat Stri Mandal

Founded by **Saralabala Devi Chaudharani** in Calcutta. It was the first All India Women Organisation.

The Indian Women's Association

Founded by **Annie Besant** in Madras (1917 AD).

Khudai Khidmatgar Movement

Started by **Khan Abdul Gaffar Khan** in NWFP (1929 AD).

Atmaram Panduran (1823 AD-1898 AD)

Atmaram Pandurang founded **Prarthana Samaj** in 1867 AD in Bombay.

The Revolt of 1857 AD

Occurred during the reign of Governor-General Lord Canning.

Causes of the Revolt

- **Political: Nana Sahib** was refused pension, as he was the adopted son of Peshwa Baji Rao II. Avadh was annexed in 1856. On charges of mal-administration, Satara, Jhansi, Nagpur and Sambhalpur were annexed owing to Doctrine of Lapse.
- **Economic:** Heavy taxation, forcibly evictions, discriminatory tariff policy against Indian products.
- **Socio-religious:** Abolition of sati in 1829 AD; legalisation of widow remarriage in 1856 AD, etc.
- **Military:** Discrimination with Indian soldiers.
- **Immediate cause:** The introduction of Enfield rifles, whose cartridges were said to have a greased cover made of beef and pork, sparked off the revolt.

Rani Laxmi Bai

Rani Laxmi Bai, nicknamed Manu was married to Raja Gangadhar Rao in 1842. The couple adopted a child in 1853 but Lord Dalhousie wished to annex Jhansi under the Doctrine of Lapse. Rani did not surrender and died fighting at Kalpi near Jhansi during the revolt of 1857

Impact of the Revolt of 1857 AD

1. In August 1857 AD, the British Parliament passed an Act which put an end to the rule of the Company. The control of the British Government in India was transferred to the British Crown.
2. The British Governor-General of India was now also given the title of Viceroy.
3. After the revolt, the British pursued the policy of **divide and rule**.

Indian National Movement

Indian National Congress (I.N.C.)

- The Indian National Union was formed in 1884 AD by A.O. Hume.

- The first session of the Indian National Congress was held at **Gokuldas Tejpal Sanskrit College** in Bombay under the presidentship of **W.C. Bannerji**.

Facts

Ist President of INC	W. C. Bannerji
Ist Woman President	Annie Besant
Ist Muslim President	Badruddin Tyabji
Ist English President	George Yuke
Gandhi became President	1924, Belgaum

The Partition of Bengal (1905) and Boycott and Swadeshi Movement (1905AD-1908 AD)

- The Partition of Bengal came into effect on 16th October, 1905 AD.
- On 7th August, 1905 AD, a resolution to boycott British goods was adopted at a meeting of the INC held in Calcutta.
- **Tilak** took the movement to different parts of India, especially in Pune and Bombay. **Ajit Singh** and **Lala Lajpat Rai** spread the Swadeshi message in Punjab and other parts of Northern India. **Syed Haider Raza** set up to agenda in Delhi. **Chidambaram Pillai** took the movement to Madras Presidency.

Formation of the Muslim League

- Set up in 1906 AD, under the leadership of Aga Khan, Nawab Salimullah of Dhaka and Nawab Mohsin-ul-Mulk.
- The extremists were led by **Bal Gangadhar Tilak**, **Lala Lajpat Rai** and **Bipin Chandra Pal** and the moderates were led by **Gopal Krishna Gokhale**.

Indian Council Act of 1909 AD or Morley-Minto Reforms

- Separate electorate introduced for Muslims.
- Non-officials to be elected indirectly. Thus, election introduced for the first time.

Ghadar Party (1913 AD)

- Formed by Lala Har Dayal, Tarak Nath Das and Sohan Singh Bhakna.
- Indian revolutionary in the United States of America and Canada had established the **Ghadar (Rebellion) Party** in 1913 AD.

Home Rule Movement (1916 AD)

The Home Rule League was pioneered on the lines of a similar movement in Ireland. The Muslim League also supported the movement.

Tilak's Home Rule Movement

The Congress Session at Allahabad in December 1921 decided to launch a **Civil Disobedience Movement**.

The Gandhian Era (1917 AD-1947 AD)

Mahatma Gandhi (1869 AD-1948 AD): Chronological Overview

In India: (1915 AD-1948 AD)

- **1915 AD:** Arrived in Bombay (India) on 9th January 1915 AD; Foundation of Satyagraha. Ashram at Kocharab near Ahmedabad (20th May). In 1917 AD, Ashram was shifted at the banks of Sabarmati.
- **1917 AD:** Gandhi entered active politics with **Champaran campaign**. Champaran Satyagraha was his first Civil Disobedience Movement in India.
- **1948 AD:** Mahatma Gandhi was shot dead by **Nathu Ram Godse** while on his way to the evening prayer meeting at **Birla House**, **New Delhi** (30th January, 1948 AD).

Main Events During the Gandhian Era

Rowlatt Act (1919 AD)

Mahatma Gandhi decided to fight against this act and he gave a call of Satyagraha on 6th April, 1919 AD. He was arrested on 8th April, 1919 AD.

Jallianwala Bagh Massacre (13th April, 1919 AD)

The arrest of **Dr. Saifuddin Kitchlu** and **Dr. Satyapal** on 10th April, 1919 AD, under the Rowlatt Act in connection with Satyagraha caused serious unrest in Punjab. A public meeting was held on 13th April, 1919 AD in a park called **Jallianwala Bagh** in **Amritsar**. As soon as the meeting started, **General Reginald Dyer** ordered indiscriminate heavy firing.

☞ **Note: Sardar Udham Singh**, an Indian patriot from Punjab, shot down General Reginald Dyer in London in 1940 AD.

Khilafat Movement (1920 AD-1922 AD)

The Ali Brothers–Mohammad Ali and **Shaukat Ali**–launched an anti-British movement in 1920 AD–the movement for the restoration of the Khilafat Movement. **Maulana Abul Kalam Azad** also led the movement. It was supported by **Mahatma** Gandhi and INC.

Non-cooperation Movement (1920 AD-1922 AD)

At the **Calcutta session** in September 1920 AD, the Congress resolved in favour of the Non-cooperation Movement and defined **Swaraj** as its ultimate aim (according to Gandhiji).

There was an attack on a local police station by angry peasants at **Chauri Chaura** in Gorakhpur district on 5th February, 1922 AD. Mahatma Gandhi, shocked by Chauri Chaura incident, withdrew the Non-Cooperation Movement on 12th February, 1922 AD.

The Swarajists

- In December 1922 AD, C.R. Das and Motilal Nehru formed Congress Khilafat Swarajya Party with C.R. Das as the President and Motilal Nehru as the Secretary.
- Madan Mohan Malaviya and Lala Lajpat Rai founded the **Independent Congress Party** later in 1933 AD. It was recognised as the Congress Nationalist Party.

Simon Commission (1927 AD)

- In 1927 AD, the British Government appointed the **Indian Statutory Commission** known popularly by its chairman Simon.
- The **Muslim League** and **Hindu Mahasabha** decided to support the Congress.
- At Lahore, Lala Lajpat Rai was severely beaten in a lathicharge and he succumbed to his injuries.

Nehru Report (1928 AD)

- Nehru report was tabled in 1928 AD by **Motilal Nehru**.
- It remains memorable as the first major Indian effort to draft a constitutional framework for India.

Dandi March/Salt Satyagraha (1930 AD)

- Along with 78 followers, Mahatma Gandhi started his famous march from **Sabarmati Ashram** on 12th March, 1930 AD for the small village **Dandi** to break the Salt Law.
- Under the leadership of Abdul Gaffar Khan, popularly known as **The Frontier Gandhi**, the Pathans organised the society of **Khudai Khidmatgars** (servants of God) known popularly as **Red Shirts**.

The Government of India Act, 1935

The Simon Commission report submitted in 1930 AD formed the basis for the Government of India Act, 1935. The Act: (i) introduced provincial autonomy; (ii) abolished dyarchy in the provinces; (iii) made ministers responsible to the legislative and federation at the centre. The Act of 1935 was unanimously rejected by the Congress.

Pakistan Resolution/Lahore Resolution (24th March, 1940 AD)

The Lahore Session of the Muslim League was held on 24th March, 1940 AD. Pakistan Resolution was passed.

August Offer/Linlithgow Offer (8th August, 1940 AD)

On this day, **Viceroy Linlithgow** came out with certain proposals known as **August Offer** declaring that the goal of the British Government was to establish **Dominion Status** in India.

Individual Civil Disobedience/ Individual Satyagraha (October 1940 AD-December 1941 AD)

The Congress Working Committee decided to individually fight disobedience on 17th October, 1940 AD. **Vinoba Bhave** was the first Satyagrahi, followed soon by many more, including **Nehru** and **Patel**.

Cripps Mission (1942 AD)

The British Government's refusal of accepting immediately the Congress demand was the cause of failure of the mission.

Quit India Movement (1942 AD)

- The All India Congress Committee met at **Bombay** on 8th August, 1942 AD. It passed the famous **Quit India** resolution and proposed to the starting of a non-violent mass struggle under **Gandhiji's leadership**.
- It is also called **Vardha Proposal** and **Leaderless Revolt**.
- His message was **'Do or Die'**.

Demand for Pakistan

- In 1930 AD, Mohammad Iqbal, for the first time, suggested that the frontier province, Sind, Baluchistan and Kashmir be made the Muslim state within the federation.
- Chaudhry Rehmat Ali coined the term **'Pakstan'** (later **'Pakistan'**).
- **Pakistan Resolution:** The Muslim League first passed the proposal of separate Pakistan in its Lahore Session in 1940 AD (called Jinnah's two-nation theory).

The Indian National Army and Subhash Chandra Bose

- The idea of Indian National Army (INA) was first conceived in Malaya by **Mohan Singh**, an Indian officer of the British Indian Army.
- In March 1942, a conference of India was held in Tokyo and **Indian Independence League** was formed.
- Subhash Chandra Bose escaped to Berlin in 1941 AD and set up **Indian League** there.
- He formed **Forward Bloc** in 1939 AD.

INA Trials

12th November, 1945 was celebrated as the INA Day.

Cabinet Mission (March-June, 1946 AD)

The Cabinet Mission, which included **Lord Pathick Lawrence Stafford Cripps** and **AV. Alexander** visited India and met the representatives of different political parties. The Mission envisaged the establishment of a Constituent Assembly to frame the constitution as well as an interim government.

Direct Action Campaign (16th August, 1946 AD): The Muslim League launched a direct action campaign on 16th August, 1946 AD, which resulted in widespread communal riots in the country.

Interim Government

- Interim Government was headed by **Jawahar Lal Nehru**.
- The **Constituent Assembly** begins its session on **9th December, 1946 AD** and Dr. Rajendra Prasad was elected its President.
- **Mountbatten** would replace Wavell as the Viceroy.

Mountbatten Plan (3rd June, 1947 AD)

- **3rd June Plan:** In case of partition, two dominions and two Constituent Assemblies would be created. The plan declared that power would be handed over by 15th August, 1947 AD.
- Mountbatten's formula was to divide India but retain maximum unity.

India Independence Act, 1947 AD

- On 18th July, 1947 AD, the British Parliament ratified the Mountbatten Plan as the **Independence of India Act, 1947**.
- The Act provided creation of two independent dominions of India and Pakistan.
- On 15th August, 1947, India got independence. Jinnah became the first Governor-General of Pakistan. India requested Mountbatten to continue as the Governor-General of India.

Governor-Generals and Viceroys

Robert Clive

Governor of Bengal during 1757 AD-1760 AD and again 1765 AD-1767 AD and established Dual Government in Bengal from 1765 AD-1772 AD.

Warren Hastings (1774 AD-1785AD)

- He became Governor of Bengal in 1772 AD and first Governor-General of Bengal in 1773 AD.
- Established India's first Supreme Court in Calcutta.

Lord Cornwallis (1786 AD-1793AD)

- He introduced Izaredari System in 1773 AD.
- He started the **permanent settlement of Bengal**.
- He created the post of **District Judge.** He is called Father of Civil Services in India.

Lord Wellesley (1798 AD-1803 AD)

- Introduced the system of Subsidiary alliance. Madras Presidency was formed during his tenure.
- In 1800 AD, he set up Fort William College in Calcutta. He was famous as Bengal Tiger.
- He brought the censorship of Press Act, 1799 AD.

Lord Minto (1807 AD-1813 AD)

- Treaty of Amritsar (1809 AD) with Ranjit Singh.
- Charter Act of 1813 AD ended the monopoly of East India Company in India.

Lord Hastings (1813 AD-1823 AD)

- Adopted the policy of intervention and war.
- Introduced the Ryotwari settlement in Madras by Thomas Munro, the Governor.

Lord William Bentinck (1828 AD-1834AD)

- Regarded as the 'Father of Modern Western Education in India'.

- Abolition of Sati in 1829 AD.
- Suppression of Thugi (1830 AD).
- Deposition of Raja of Mysore and annexation of his territories (1831 AD).
- He was the First Governor-General of India.

Lord Ellenborough (1842 AD-1844 AD)

Abolished slavery (1843 AD).

Lord Dalhousie (1848 AD-1856 AD)

- Abolished Titles and pensions, Widow Remarriage Act (1856 AD).
- Started the first railway line in 1853 AD; Started electric telegraph service. Laid the basis of the modern Postal System (1854 AD); A separate public works department was set up for the first time.

Lord Canning (1856 AD-1858AD)

- The last Governor General of East India Company
- He withdrew Doctrine of Lapse.

Lord Canning (1858 AD-1862AD)

The Indian Councils Act of 1861 AD was passed; Indian Penal Code of Criminal Procedure (1859 AD) was passed; The Indian High Court Act (1861 AD) was enacted; Income-tax was introduced for the first time in 1858 AD; The Universities of Calcutta, Bombay and Madras founded in 1857 AD.

Sir Johan Lawrence (1864 AD-1869 AD):

High Courts were established at Calcutta Bombay and Madras in 1865 AD.

Lord Mayo (1869 AD-1872 AD)

- He established the Department of Agriculture and Commerce.
- In 1872 AD, first Census was done in India.
- He was the only **Viceroy to be murdered** in office by a convict in the Andaman in 1872 AD.

Lord Lytton (1876 AD-1880 AD)

- Most infamous Governor-General; Arranged the Grand Darbar in Delhi; Royal Title Act (1876 AD) and Queen Victoria was declared as the Kaisari Hind.
- The infamous **Vernacular Press Act** (1878 AD) and lowered the maximum age of ICS from 21 to 19 years.

Lord Ripon (1880 AD-1884 AD)

- He was famously known as "Father of Local Self-Government".
- First Official Census in India (1881 AD).
- Appointed **Hunter Commission** for education reforms in 1882AD.

Lord Dufferin (1884 AD-1888AD)

- Formation of **Indian National Congress** (INC) in 1885 AD.
- Dufferin called INC as 'microscopic minority'.

Lord Curzon (1899 AD-1905AD)

- Appointed a Police Commission in 1902 AD under Andrew Frazer.
- Indian Universities Act passed in 1904 AD.
- Famine Commission under MacDonnell.

Lord Minto II (1905 AD-1910AD)

Swadeshi Movement (1905 AD-1908 AD); Foundation of the Muslim League, 1906 AD; Surat session and split in the Congress (1907 AD).

Lord Hardinge (1910 AD-1916AD)

- Annulment of the Partition of Bengal (1911), Transfer of capital from Calcutta to Delhi (1911); Delhi Darbar and Coronation of King George V and Queen Mary (1911).
- In 1911, Bihar and Orissa separated from Bengal and, became a new state.

Lord Chelmsford (1916 AD-1921 AD)

Home Rule Movement launched by Tilak and Annie Besant (1916); Lucknow Pact between Congress and Muslim League (1916); Arrival of Mahatma Gandhi in India (1915); Champaran Satyagraha (1917); Repressive Rowlatt Act (1919); Jallianwala Bagh Massacre (April 13, 1919). Khilafat Movement (1920–1922); Non-Cooperation Movement (1920–1922).

Lord Reading (1921 AD-1926AD)

- Rowlatt Act was repealed along with Press Act of 1910.
- Chauri-Chaura incident and withdrawal of Non-Cooperation Movement.
- Formation of Swaraj Party by CR Das and Motilal Nehru (1923).
- Kakori Train Conspiracy (1925).
- Lee Commission (1924) for public services.
- **RSS** founded in 1925.

Lord Irwin (1926 AD-1931 AD)

- Simon Commission visited India in 1928.
- Nehru Report, 1928.
- Lahore Session of the Congress, (1929) and Poorna Swaraj, declaration.
- Civil Disobedience Movement, 1930 started with.
- **Dandi March** (12 March 1930).
- Gandhi-Irwin Pact, 5 March 1931.
- Jawaharlal Nehru and Subhash Chandra Bose founded **Independence of India League.**

Lord Willingdon (1931 AD-1936AD)

Civil Disobedience Movement (1932); Announcement of MacDonald. Communal Award (1932); Foundation of Congress Socialist Party–CSP (1934); Burma Separated from India (1935), All India Kisan Sabha (1936).

Lord Linlithgow (1934 AD-1944AD)

- First General Election (1936–37) Congress Ministries.
- Deliverance day by Muslim League 1939.
- Lahore Resolution of Muslim League (1940) demand of Pakistan.
- August Offer, 1940.
- Cripps Mission, 1942.
- Quit India Movement, 1942.
- "Divide and Quit" at the Karachi Session (1940).
- In Haripura Session (1939) of Congress complete Independence was declared.

Governor Generals of Free India (1947 AD-1950 AD)

Lord Mountbatten (1947–1948)

The first Governor General of free Indian); Murder of Gandhi (Jan. 30, 1948).

C. Rajagopalachari (June 1948–January 25, 1950)

The last Governor General of free India; The only Indian Governor General.

Exercise

1. In which Indian Religion, there are 24 Tirthankaras?
(a) Jainism (b) Buddhism
(c) Hinduism (d) Sikhism

2. The oldest rock-cut architecture is found in ____.
(a) Rajasthan (b) Bihar
(c) Karnataka (d) Mizoram

3. Rashtrapati Bhavan was built in ____.
(a) 1852 (b) 1910
(c) 1947 (d) 1986

4. Santhara is a religious ritual of ____ community.
(a) Sikhs (b) Jews
(c) Jain (d) Buddhists

5. Battle of Haldighati was fought in the year ____.
(a) 1764 (b) 1526
(c) 1576 (d) 1857

6. Group of Monuments at Hampi is in ____.
(a) Karnataka
(b) Madhya Pradesh
(c) Maharashtra
(d) Rajasthan

7. Chang Lo is a folk dance of ____.
(a) Arunachal Pradesh
(b) Punjab
(c) Assam
(d) Nagaland

8. Chanakya was the chief advisor of ____.
(a) Babur
(b) Chandragupta Maurya
(c) Akbar
(d) Kautilya

9. Battle of Haldighati in 1576 was fought between Akbar and ____.
(a) Sher Shah
(b) Maharana Pratap
(c) Hemu Vikramaditya
(d) Nader Shah

10. Gandhi Irwin pact happened in which year?
(a) 1905 (b) 1931
(c) 1947 (d) 1942

11. In 1739, who defeated the Mughal army at the Battle of Karnal?
(a) Nader Shah
(b) Genghis Khan
(c) Hemu Vikramaditya
(d) Bajirao I

12. The Red Fort (Delhi) was built by ____.
(a) Babur (b) British
(c) Shah Jahan (d) Aurangzeb

13. Whom did Akbar defeat in the 2nd battle of Panipat in 1556?
(a) Genghis Khan
(b) Nader Shah
(c) Hemu Vikramaditya
(d) Bajirao I

14. Aurangzeb, the Mughal Emperor died in?
(a) 1507 (b) 1607
(c) 1707 (d) 1807

15. Shiva cave is located in ____.
(a) Ajanta Caves
(b) Ellora Caves
(c) Elephanta Caves
(d) Badami Caves

16. Rock Shelters of Bhimbetka is in ____.
(a) Maharashtra
(b) Himachal Pradesh
(c) Karnataka
(d) Madhya Pradesh

17. Before its Independence, Bangladesh was part of ____.
(a) India
(b) China
(c) Pakistan
(d) United Kingdom

18. Humayun was born in the year ____.
(a) 1508 (b) 1608
(c) 1708 (d) 1808

19. Ashoka converted to which religion after the Kalinga war?
(a) Jainism (b) Buddhism
(c) Christianity (d) Judaism

20. Gandhi Ji started the Non-Cooperation Movement in ____.
(a) 1880 (b) 1900
(c) 1920 (d) 1940

21. Chhatrapati Shivaji Terminus station was designed by
(a) Frederick William Stevens
(b) Santiago Calatrava
(c) Fazlur Rahman Khan
(d) Frei Otto

22. Chhatrapati Sambhaji (1680-1688 AD) was the ruler of which dynasty?
(a) Maratha (b) Nanda
(c) Haryanka (d) Maurya

23. Birbal was an advisor in the court of ____.
(a) Babur (b) Akbar
(c) Aurangzeb (d) Jahangir

24. Humayun's Tomb is located in ___.
(a) Delhi (b) Agra
(c) Gwalior (d) Jaipur

25. The decision to effect the Partition of Bengal was announced in 1905 by
(a) Lord William Bentinck
(b) Lord Mountbatten
(c) Warren Hastings
(d) Lord Curzon

26. Who set up the Sabarmati Ashram in Ahmedabad?
(a) Subhash Chandra Bose
(b) Mohandas Gandhi
(c) Jawaharlal Nehru
(d) Sarojini Naidu

27. ____ is a depiction of the Hindu God Shiva as the cosmic dancer who performs his divine dance called Tandavam.
(a) Murugan (b) Nataraja
(c) Vishnu (d) Venkateshwar

28. Which among the following games was very popular in ancient India?
(a) Chess (b) Cricket
(c) Hockey (d) Football

29. Ashoka The Great (273-232 B.C.) was the ruler of which dynasty?
(a) Mewar (b) Mughal
(c) Maurya (d) Peshwas

30. Indus Valley Civilization was a __ age civilization.
(a) Silver (b) Tin
(c) Gold (d) Bronze

31. To whom did Akbar gave the title Mian?
(a) Raja Todar Mal
(b) Man Singh I
(c) Birbal
(d) Tansen

32. Churches and Convents of Goa were built by
(a) British (b) Dutch
(c) Portuguese (d) Mughals

33. Ghatotkacha (who ruled in the years 290-305 B.C.) was a king from which dynasty?
(a) Gupta Dynasty
(b) Kanva Dynasty
(c) Shunga Dynasty
(d) Maurya Dynasty

34. Who are credited to a large extent for ending the Mughal rule in India?
(a) Mauryas (b) Cholas
(c) Guptas (d) Marathas

35. Ajanta Caves is in ____.
(a) Maharashtra
(b) Himachal Pradesh
(c) Karnataka
(d) Madhya Pradesh

36. In 1617 the British East India Company was given permission by ____ to trade in India.
(a) Babur (b) Akbar
(c) Aurangzeb (d) Jahangir

37. Who built the Group of Monuments at Pattadakal?
(a) Chola Kings
(b) Pallava Kings
(c) Chera Kings
(d) Chalukya Kings

38. The Kalinga war was fought in ____.
(a) 161 BC (b) 261 BC
(c) 361 BC (d) 461 BC

39. Tipu Sultan was also known as the Lion of ____.
(a) Bangalore (b) Delhi
(c) Kochi (d) Mysore

40. Who built the Buddhist Monuments at Sanchi?
(a) Mughal Dynasty
(b) Maurya Dynasty
(c) Gupta Dynasty
(d) Chola Dynasty

41. When was the battle of Haldighati fought?
(a) 1776 (b) 1676
(c) 1576 (d) 1476

42. In 1498, which Portuguese explorer discovered a new sea route from Europe to India?
(a) Vasco da Gama
(b) Christopher Columbus
(c) Sir Francis Drake
(d) John Cabot

43. Buland Darwaza is the main entrance to the palace at ____.
(a) Amer Fort
(b) Gwalior Fort
(c) Fatehpur Sikri
(d) Agra Fort

44. Who was the first ruler of Pala dynasty?
(a) Gopala
(b) Vivyanathan
(c) Dharmapala
(d) Bhaskaran

45. Which empire is regarded as the Golden Age of Hinduism?
(a) Maurya (b) Mughal
(c) Gupta (d) Chola

46. ____ is a collection of architectural astronomical instruments, built by Maharaja Jai Singh II.
(a) Jantar Mantar, Delhi
(b) Group of Monuments at Hampi
(c) Group of Monuments at Pattadakal
(d) Nalanda, Bihar

47. Tripitakas are sacred books of ____.
(a) Sikhs (b) Jews
(c) Buddhists (d) Muslims

48. Bahadur Shah I (1707-1712 AD) was the ruler of which dynasty?
(a) Nanda (b) Maurya
(c) Mughal (d) Haryanka

49. Khas Mahal and the Shish Mahal are built in which World Heritage Monument?
(a) Humayun's Tomb
(b) Mahabodhi Temple Complex
(c) Qutub Minar
(d) Agra Fort

50. Diwane-i-khas is in which of these monuments?
(a) Humayun's Tomb
(b) Mahabodhi Temple Complex
(c) Qutub Minar
(d) Red Fort Complex

51. During the Independence Movement, Subhash Chandra Bose revamped the Indian National ____.
(a) Navy (b) Army
(c) Defence (d) Air Force

52. Aurangzeb was the son of ____.
(a) Babur (b) Humayun
(c) Akbar (d) Shah Jahan

53. Who built the Group of Monuments at Mahabalipuram?
(a) Chola Kings
(b) Pallava Kings
(c) Chera Kings
(d) Chalukya Kings

54. Bimbisara was the king of which dynasty?
(a) Haryanka (b) Maurya
(c) Shunga (d) Nanda

55. World War I started in the year
(a) 1914 (b) 1919
(c) 1939 (d) 1945

56. Moti Masjid is situated in which of these World Heritage Sites?
(a) Humayun's Tomb
(b) Mahabodhi Temple Complex
(c) Qutub Minar
(d) Red Fort Complex

57. Who was the trusted General of the Mughal emperor Akbar?
(a) Raja Todar Mal
(b) Man Singh I
(c) Birbal
(d) Tansen

58. Who was the trusted General of the Mughal emperor Akbar?
(a) Raja Todar Mal
(b) Man Singh I
(c) Birbal
(d) Tansen

59. Mausoleum (Dargah) of Salim Chishti is situated in ____.
(a) Humayun's Tomb
(b) Fatehpur Sikri
(c) Gwlior Fort
(d) Agra Fort

60. Qutub Minar is located in ____.
(a) Delhi (b) Ghaziabad
(c) Noida (d) Gurugram

61. Bajirao I (1720-1740 AD) was the ruler of which dynasty?
(a) Nanda (b) Peshwas
(c) Haryanka (d) Maurya

62. Which of these railway stations is a World Heritage Site?
(a) Kharagpur Railway Station
(b) Howrah Station
(c) Chhatrapati Shivaji Terminus
(d) Kanpur Central

63. Akbar's regime, ____ was the military head.
(a) Sultan Ahmed Fawad
(b) Suri Moja
(c) Mir Khaas
(d) Mir Bakshi

64. Who pioneered the guerrilla warfare methods?
(a) Babur
(b) Akbar
(c) Shivaji
(d) Bajirao Peshwa

65. Ajanta Caves in Maharashtra have rock-cut cave monuments of which religion?
(a) Sikhism (b) Buddhism
(c) Christianity (d) Hinduism

66. Whose reign in Indian History is called the Golden Age of India?
(a) Mughal Empire
(b) Maratha Empire
(c) Gupta Empire
(d) Maurya Empire

67. Who was the second woman to become the president of the Indian National Congress in 1925 and the first Indian woman to do so?
(a) Vijaylakshmi Pandit
(b) Sarojini Naidu
(c) Padmaja Naidu
(d) Fathima Bibi

68. Which caves is a cultural mix of religious arts of Buddhism, Hinduism and Jainism?
(a) Ajanta (b) Ellora
(c) Elephanta (d) Badami

69. Which World Heritage Monument has been acclaimed as the "Necropolis of the Mughal dynasty"?
(a) Humayun's Tomb
(b) Mahabodhi Temple Complex
(c) Qutub Minar
(d) Red Fort Complex

70. Who was first Viceroy and Governor-General of pre-independence era?
(a) Warren Hastings
(b) Lord William Bentinck
(c) Lord Mountbatten
(d) Lord Canning

71. Jahangir was the son of ____.
(a) Babur (b) Humayun
(c) Akbar (d) Shah Jahan

72. ____ caves are a network of sculpted caves located in Mumbai Harbour.
(a) Ajanta (b) Ellora
(c) Elephanta (d) Badami

73. The Renaissance is a period in Europe, from the ____.
(a) 18th to the 20th century
(b) 14th to the 17th century
(c) 11th to the 13th century
(d) 7th to the 10th century

74. Aurangzeb (1658-1707 AD) was the ruler of which dynasty?
(a) Nanda (b) Mughal
(c) Maurya (d) Haryanka

75. Which world heritage site comprises of the tomb of Iltutmish?
(a) Humayun's Tomb
(b) Mahabodhi Temple Complex
(c) Qutub Minar
(d) Red Fort Complex

76. Khajuraho Group of monuments are attributed to which dynasty?
(a) Chandela (b) Mughal
(c) Maurya (d) Shunga

77. Which world heritage site comprises of the Alai Darwaza Gate?
(a) Humayun's Tomb
(b) Mahabodhi Temple Complex
(c) Qutub Minar
(d) Red Fort Complex

78. Babur (1526-1530 AD) was the ruler of which dynasty?
(a) Mughal (b) Nanda
(c) Maurya (d) Haryanka

79. Who built Jodhpur Fort?
(a) Guru Ramdas
(b) Shah Jahan
(c) Rao Jodhaji
(d) Mahatma Gandhi

80. Battle of Panipat was fought in the year ____.
(a) 1764 (b) 1757
(c) 1526 (d) 1857

81. Noor Jahan was wife of which Mughal Emperor?
(a) Akbar (b) Aurangzeb
(c) Jahangir (d) Shah Jahan

82. Battle of Tarain was fought in the year ____?
(a) 1526 (b) 1757
(c) 1191 (d) 1857

83. Garden inside the Taj Mahal is known as ____.
(a) Mughal Garden
(b) Taj Bageecha
(c) Taj Mahal Garden
(d) Mahal Bageecha

84. Who started the Home Rule League?
(a) Bal Gangadhar Tilak
(b) Rajendra Prasad
(c) Mahatma Gandhi
(d) Jawahar Lal Nehru

85. The name by which Ashoka is generally referred to in his inscription is ____?
(a) Chakravarti (b) Dharmadeva
(c) Priyadarshi (d) Dharmakrit

86. Which temple is built in the form of the chariot of Surya, the Sun God with 24 wheels?
(a) Soorya Narayana Temple
(b) Dakshinaraka Temple
(c) Surya Pahar Temple
(d) Konark Sun Temple

87. The battle of Tarain was fought between Prithviraj Chauhan and __.
(a) Mahmood Gaznabi
(b) Muhammad Ghori
(c) Babar
(d) Humayun

88. Isfahan, the Persian Capital is said to have provided the inspiration to build which of these monuments?
(a) Humayun's Tomb
(b) Mahabodhi Temple Complex
(c) Qutub Minar
(d) Red Fort Complex

89. Akbar (1556-1605 AD) was the ruler of which dynasty?
(a) Nanda (b) Maurya
(c) Mughal (d) Haryanka

90. The Bibi Ka Maqbara is a tomb located in ____. It was built by Azam Shah, son of Aurangzeb, in 1678.
(a) Hyderabad (b) Aurangabad
(c) Lucknow (d) Allahabad

91. Battle of Kanauj was fought in the year ____.
(a) 1764 (b) 1526
(c) 1540 (d) 1857

92. Ashoka was an emperor of the ____Dynasty.
(a) Mughal (b) Chola
(c) Maurya (d) Gupta

93. Which Mughal emperor imprisoned his father and executed his brother?
(a) Babur (b) Humayun
(c) Aurangzeb (d) Shah Alam II

94. Humayun's Tomb was built by ____.
(a) Humayun
(b) Hamida Banu Begum
(c) Babur
(d) Akbar

95. Who built Sabarmati Ashram?
(a) Guru Ramdas
(b) Shah Jahan
(c) Rao Jodhaji
(d) Mahatma Gandhi

96. From which monument, Gautama Buddha propagated his divine knowledge of Buddhism to the world?
(a) Humayun's Tomb
(b) Mahabodhi Temple Complex
(c) Qutub Minar
(d) Red Fort Complex

97. Jahangir was born in the year ____.
(a) 1569 (b) 1669
(c) 1769 (d) 1869

98. Bahadur Shah (First) was born in the year ____.
(a) 1543 (b) 1643
(c) 1743 (d) 1843

Answers

1. (a)	**2.** (b)	**3.** (b)	**4.** (c)	**5.** (c)	**6.** (a)	**7.** (d)	**8.** (b)	**9.** (b)	**10.** (b)
11. (a)	**12.** (c)	**13.** (c)	**14.** (c)	**15.** (c)	**16.** (d)	**17.** (c)	**18.** (a)	**19.** (b)	**20.** (c)
21. (a)	**22.** (a)	**23.** (b)	**24.** (a)	**25.** (d)	**26.** (b)	**27.** (b)	**28.** (a)	**29.** (c)	**30.** (d)
31. (d)	**32.** (c)	**33.** (a)	**34.** (d)	**35.** (a)	**36.** (d)	**37.** (d)	**38.** (b)	**39.** (d)	**40.** (b)
41. (c)	**42.** (a)	**43.** (c)	**44.** (c)	**45.** (b)	**46.** (b)	**47.** (a)	**48.** (c)	**49.** (d)	**50.** (d)
51. (b)	**52.** (d)	**53.** (b)	**54.** (a)	**55.** (a)	**56.** (d)	**57.** (b)	**58.** (b)	**59.** (b)	**60.** (a)
61. (b)	**62.** (c)	**63.** (d)	**64.** (c)	**65.** (b)	**66.** (c)	**67.** (b)	**68.** (b)	**69.** (a)	**70.** (d)
71. (c)	**72.** (c)	**73.** (b)	**74.** (b)	**75.** (c)	**76.** (a)	**77.** (c)	**78.** (a)	**79.** (c)	**80.** (c)
81. (c)	**82.** (c)	**83.** (a)	**84.** (a)	**85.** (c)	**86.** (d)	**87.** (b)	**88.** (d)	**89.** (c)	**90.** (b)
91. (c)	**92.** (c)	**93.** (c)	**94.** (b)	**95.** (d)	**96.** (a)	**97.** (a)	**98.** (b)		

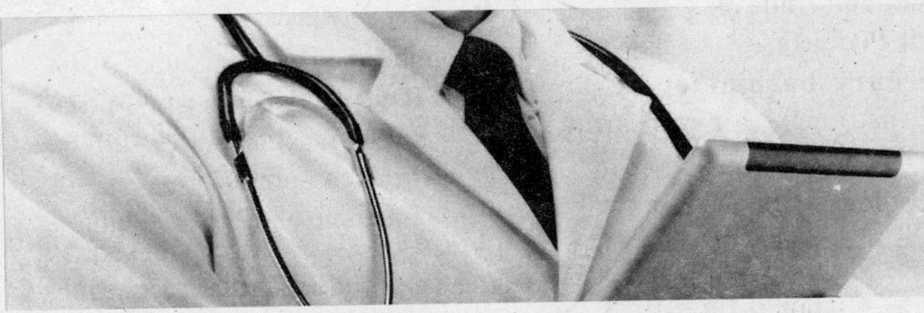

GEOGRAPHY

Universe

- The universe comprises billions of galaxies. The galaxies are made up of millions of stars held together by the force of gravity and these stars account for most of the masses of the galaxy.

Stars

- Stars are made of hot burning gases.
- They emit light of their own and are very large and very hot.
- Light takes about 4.3 years to reach us from the next nearest star **Proxima Centauri**.

The Sun

- It is the nearest star to the earth.
- Its diameter is 14 lakh km.
- It is composed of 71% Hydrogen, 26.5% helium and 2.5% other elements.

The Earth

- The Earth is 23½° tilted on its axis and, thus, makes 66½° angle.
- It takes 23 hours 56 minutes and 4.091 seconds to rotate on its axis.
- Earth is known as the **"watery planet"** or the **"blue planet"**.
- Earth is the only known planet which provides sustenance of life on it.

The Moon

- The Moon is the only satellite of the earth.
- It has diameter of 3475 km and its circumference is 10864 km while its orbit is elliptical.

Specifics of the Planets	
Biggest planet	Jupiter
Biggest Satellite	Ganymede
Blue planet	Earth
Green planet	Uranus
Brightest planet	Venus
Brightest star (outside solar system)	Sirius (Dog Star)
Closest star of solar system	Proxima Centauri
Coldest planet	Neptune
Evening star	Venus
Farthest planet from Sun	Neptune
Planet with maximum number of satellites	Jupiter
Hottest planet	Venus
Densest planet	Earth
Morning star	Venus
Nearest planet to Earth	Venus
Nearest planet to Sun	Mercury
Red planet	Mars
Smallest planet	Mercury
Earth twin	Venus

Meteors and Meteorites

- Meteors and Meteorites are also called shooting stars.
- When meteors are large and do not burn up completely, they land on the earth's surface and are known as **Meteorites**.

Biosphere

The part of the earth where life exists is called the **Biosphere** ('bios' means 'life').

Lithosphere

- The uppermost layer of the earth's crust which is capable of supporting life is called Lithosphere.
- The Lithosphere (or land) covers two-sevenths or 29.22% of the total surface area of the earth.

Hydrosphere

Hydrosphere (or sea) covers 70.70% of the total surface area of the earth.

Latitude

Latitude is the angular distance of a point on the earth surface from the centre of earth, measured in degree. These lines are called parallels of latitude and on the globe they are circles.

Longitude

- Longitude is the angular distance of a point on the earth surface along the equator, east or west from the **Prime Meridian.**
- Prime Meridian is the semi-circle from pole to pole, from which all the other meridians radiate Eastwards and Westwards up to 180°.
- 180° meridian **(International Date Line)** is exactly opposite to the Prime Meridian. Such points are called anti-pedal points.

Local Time (LT) and Time Zones

- The Indian Government has accepted the meridian of 82.5 degree east for standard time, which is 5 hrs. 30 mins. ahead of the Greenwich Mean Time.
- Russia has as many as 11 time zones.
- Both USA and Canada have five time zones.

The Date Line and Universal Time (UT)

- It is the 180 degree meridian running over the Pacific Ocean, deviating at Aleutian Island, Fiji, Samoa and Gilbert Island.

The international date line has been established most of it following the 180th meridian–where by common agreement, whenever we cross it the date advances one day (going west) or goes back one day (going east).

- The line passes the **Bering Strait** between Alaska and Siberia.

Longest day in the Northern hemisphere	21 June
Shortest day in the Northern hemisphere	22 December
Equal day and night in the Northern hemisphere	21 March and 23 September
Longest day in the Southern hemisphere	22 December
Shortest day in Southern hemisphere	21 June
Equal day and night in the Southern hemisphere	21 March and 23 September

Earthquakes

- The sudden tremors or shaking of the earth's crust is called an **earthquake.**
- **'Seismology'** deals with the study of earthquake.
- **'Richter scale'** and **'Mercalli scale'** are the instruments to measure record the magnitude and the **intensity** of an earthquake respectively.

Atmosphere

The atmosphere extends to about 1000 km from the surface of the earth. But 99% of the total mass of the atmosphere is found within 32 km.

Composition of the Atmosphere

(i) Nitrogen–78%, (ii) Oxygen–21%, (iii) Argon–0.93%, (iv) Carbon dioxide–0.03%, (v) Neon–0.0018%, (vi) Helium–0.0005%, (vii). Ozone–0.006%, (viii) Hydrogen–0.0005%.

Structure of the Atmosphere

There are five distinct layers of the atmosphere– (a) Troposphere, (b) Stratosphere, (c) Mesosphere, (d) Thermosphere, and (e) Exosphere.

Measurement and Units of Atmospheric Pressure

- The **mercury barometer** is the standard instrument for measuring atmospheric pressure.
- **Standard sea level pressure is 76 km of 29.92 inches on this scale.**
- Orica atmospheric pressure (76 cm of mercury) = 760 mm of Hg = 1013.25 millibars (mb).

Winds

- Wind is the movement of air caused by the uneven heating of the earth by the sun.
- The air moves from high pressure to low pressure.
- The imaginary line joining the points having same pressure is called **isobars.**

Humidity

- Humidity of air refers to the contents of the water vapour present in the air at a particular time and place.
- Humidity is measured by an instrument called hygrometer.

Forests

They are of the following types:

(a) **Tropical Evergreen Rain Forests:** The leaves of trees in such forests are very wide. Examples: Red wood, palm, etc.

(b) **Tropical Semi-Deciduous Forests:** Such forests receive rainfall less than 150 cms. Saagwan, saal, bamboo, etc. are found in such forests.

(c) **Tundra Forests:** Such forests are covered with snow. Only Mosses, a few sledges and Lichens grow here in the summer.

Famous Grassland of the world

Grassland		Countries
Steppe	–	Eurasis
Prairie	–	U.S.A.
Pampas	–	Argentina
Veld	–	South Africa
Downs	–	Australia

Some Important Facts

World Continents

Continents	Biggest Country	Highest Peak	Longest River
Asia	China	Mt. Everest (8850 m)	Yangtze Kiang
Africa	Sudan	Mt. Kilimanjaro (5895 m)	Nile
Australia	Australia	Mt. Kosciuszko (2228 m)	Darling
Antarctica		Vinson Massif (5140 m)	
North America	Canada	Mt. Mckinley (6194 m)	Mississippi Missouri
South America	Brazil	Mt. Aconcagua (6960 m)	Amazon
Europe	Russia	Mt. Elbrus (5642 m)	Ob

Major Rivers of the World

River	Origin	Length (m)	Falls in
Nile	Victoria Lake	6,650	Mediterranean Sea
Amazon	Andes (Peru)	6,428	Atlantic Ocean
Yangtze	Tibetan Kiang Plateau	6,300	China Sea
Mississippi Missouri	Itaska Lake (USA)	6,275	Gulf of Mexico (USA)
Yenisei	Tannu-Ola Mts.	5,539	Arctic Ocean
Huang Ho	Kunlun Mts.	5,464	Gulf of Chibli
Ob	Altai Mts.	5,410	Russia Gulf of Ob
Congo	Lualaba and Luapula rivers	4,700	Atlantic Ocean
Amur	North-east	4,444	China Sea of Okhotsk
Lena	Baikal Mts.	4,400	Laptev Sea
Mekong	Tibetan Highlands	4,350	South China Sea
Mackenzie	Great Slave Lake	4,241	Beaufort Sea
Niger	Guinea	4,200	Gulf of Guinea

Major Lakes of the World

Highest Lake	Lake Titicaca in Bolivia
Largest Saline Water Lake	Lake Caspian Sea
Deepest Lake	Lake Baikal in Siberia
Largest Lake	Caspian Sea
Largest Fresh Water Lake	Lake Superior
India's Largest Lake	Chilka Lake in Orissa

Oceans of the World

Oceans	Area (sq.km)	Greatest Depth
Pacific	16,62,40,000	Mariana Trench
Atlantic	8,65,60,000	Puerto Rico Trench
Indian	7,34,30,000	Java Trench
Arctic	1,32,30,000	–
Antarctic/Southern	2,03,30,000.	South Sandwich Trench

Important Cities on River Banks (World)

City	River	Country
Amsterdam	Amsel	Netherlands
Ankara	Kazil	Turkey
Bangkok	Chao Praya	Thailand
Basra	Eupharates and Tigris	Iraq
Baghdad	Tigris	Iraq
Berlin	Spree	Germany
Bonn	Rhine	Germany
Budapest	Danube	Hungary
Bristol	Avon	UK
Buenos Aires	Laplata	Argentina
Chittagong	Majyani	Bangladesh
Canton	Si-Kiang	China
Cairo	Nile	Egypt
Chung King	Yang-tse-king	China
Cologne	Rhine	Germany
Dresden	Elbe	Germany
Hamburg	Elbe	Germany
Kabul	Kabul	Afghanistan
Karachi	Indus	Pakistan
Khartoum	Confluence of Blue and White Nile	Sudan
Lahore	Ravi	Pakistan
Leningrad	Neva	Russia
Lisbon	Tagus	Portugal
London	Thames	England
Moscow	Moskva	Russia
Montreal	St. Lawrence	Canada
New Orleans	Mississipi	USA
New York	Hudson	USA
Ottawa	Ottawa	Canada
Paris	Seine	France
Perth	Swan	Australia
Prague	Vitava	Czech Republic
Rome	Tiber	Italy
Rotterdam	New Mass	The Netherlands

Stalingrad	Volga	Russia
Sidney	Darling	Australia
Tokyo	Arakava	Japan
Vienna	Danube	Austria
Warsaw	Vistula	Poland
Washington DC	Potomac	USA
Yangoon	Irrawaddy	Myanmar

Important Boundaries

Durand Line	Pakistan and Afghanistan
MacMohan Line	India and China
Radcliffe Line	India and Pakistan
Maginot Line	France and Germany
Oder Niesse Line	Germany and Poland
Hindenberg Line	Poland and Germany (at the time of First World War)
38th Parallel	North and South Korea
49th Parallel	USA and Canada

Geography of India

The Indian Subcontinent

Mainland of the Indian Subcontinent, comprising India, Pakistan, Bangladesh, Nepal, and Bhutan extends between 8°4'N and 37°9'N latitudes and between 68°7'E and 97°15'E longitudes.

Size and Extent of Subcontinent

- From North to South this subcontinent stretches over 3,200 km and from east to west it is 3,000 km. 82°30' E meridian helps in calculating the Indian Standard Time (IST) which is 5 hours 30 minutes ahead of the Greenwich Mean Time (GMT).
- This very meridian (82½°E) dictates time in Sri Lanka and Nepal also.

Political Divisions of India

India is divided into 29 States and 7 Union Territories.

Basic information

- Latitudinal extent: 8°4' North to 37°6' North.
- Longitudinal extent: 68°7' East to 97°25' East.
- North south extent: 3214 km.
- East west extent: 2933 km.
- Land frontiers: 15200 km.
- Total coastline: 7516.6 km.
- Number of states: 29.
- Number of union territories: 7.
- Land neighbours (7): Pakistan, Afghanistan, China, Nepal, Bhutan, Bangladesh and Myanmar.
- State with longest coastline: Gujarat.
- Active volcano: Barren Island in Andaman and nicobar.
- Southernmost point; Indira point in great Nicobar.
- Southernmost tip main land: Kanyakumari.
- Northernmost point: Indira Col.
- Westenmost point: West of ghaur mota in Gujarat
- Easternmost point: Kibithu in Arunachal Pradesh.
- The Tropic of Cancer (23½° N) passes through the middle of the country. The location of the country is in the northern and the eastern hemispheres.

Indian states situated on the border

Country	Indian States
Pakistan (4)	Gujarat, Rajasthan, Punjab and Jammu and Kashmir
Afghanistan (1)	Jammu and Kashmir
China (5)	Jammu and Kashmir, Uttrakhand, Himachal Pradesh, Sikkim and Arunachal Pradesh
Nepal (5)	Uttar Pradesh, Uttrakhand, Bihar, West Bengal, Sikkim
Bhutan (4)	Sikkim, West Bengal, Assam and Arunachal Pradesh
Bangladesh (5)	West Bengal, Assam, Meghalaya, Tripura and Mizoram

Size of India (In Terms of Area and Population)

- India is the **seventh largest country** (in terms of area) in the world.
- India ranks as the **second largest country** in terms of population (next to China only).
- India contains about one-sixth of the total population of the world.

Physical Features

- Indian subcontinent can be divided into following physical divisions:
  - The Great Mountain wall of the North.
  - The Great Northern Plains.
  - The Great Peninsular Plateau.
  - The Coastal Plains.
  - The Great Indian Desert.
  - The Island Groups.

Himalayas

- Himalayas are young fold mountains of tertiary period, which were folded over Tethys Sea due to inter-continental collision.
- They stretch from the Indus River in the West to the Brahmaputra River in the East.
- The Himalayas, the highest mountain wall of the world, are situated on the northern boundary of India like an arc.
- Mount Everest, the highest peak in the world, lies in these mountains in Nepal.
- The total length is about 2500 km with verying width 240 to 320 km and a total area of 5000 km^2.

Divisions of the Himalayas

The Himalayas consist of three parallel mountain ranges: (i) The Greater Himalayas (ii) The Lesser Himalayas and (iii) The Outer Himalayas.

Location	Important Passes
Jammu and Kashmir	Burzi-La, Joji-La Karakorm Banihal Rohtang
Himachal Pradesh	Bara La, Cha-La, Shipki-La
Uttarakhand	Niti-La, Lipu-Lekh-La
Sikkim	Jelep-La, Nathu-La
Arunachal Pradesh	Bomdi-La

The Great Peninsular Plateau

- It is composed of old cystallin igneous and metamorphic rocks.
- It covers a total of 16000 km^2.
- Narmada which flows through a rift valley divides the region into two parts— the central highland in the north and the deccan plateau in the south.

Eastern Ghats

It comprises the discontinuous and low hills that are highly eroded by the rivers such as the Mahanadi, the Godavari, the Krishna, the Cauvery, etc.

Western Ghats

Western Ghats are locally known by different names such as Sahyadri in Maharashtra, Nilgiri hills in Karnataka and Tamil Nadu and Annamalai hills, Cardamom hills in Kerala.

The Coastal Plains

Narrow steeps of flat land on eastern and western coasts are known as the East Coastal Plain and the West Coastal Plain respectively.

The Great Indian Desert

- It lies to the west of the Aravali range.
- It is in the rain shadow area of the Bay of Bengal current.

Important River Valley Projects of India

Bhakra Nangal Project	On Satluj in Punjab. Highest in India. Height 226m. Reservoir is called Gobind Sagar Lake.
Mandi Project	On Beas in H.P.
Chambal Valley Project	On Chambal in M.P. and Rajasthan. 3 dams are there: Gandhi Sagar dam, Rana Pratap Sagar dam and Jawahar Sagar dam
Damodar Valley Project	On Damodar in Jharkhand. Based on Tennessee Valley Project, USA
Hirakud Project	On Mahanadi in Orissa. World's longest dam: 4,801 m
Rihand Project	On Son in Mirzapur. Reservoir is called Govind Vallabh Pant Reservoir
Kosi Project	On Kosi in N. Bihar
Mayurakshi Project	On Mayurakshi in W.B.
Kakrapara Project	On Tapi in Gujarat
Nizamsagar Project	On Manjra in A.P.
Nagarjuna Sagar Project	On Krishna in A.P.
Tungabhadra Project	On Tungabhadra in A.P. and Karnataka
Shivasamudram Project	On Cauvery in Karnataka
Tata Hydel Scheme	On Bhima in Maharashtra
Sharavathi Hydel Project	On Jog Falls in Karnataka
Farakka Project	On Ganga in W.B. Apart from power and irrigation, it helps to remove silt for easy navigation
Ukai Project	On Tapti in Gujarat
Mahi Project	On Mahi in Gujarat
Salal Project	On Chenab in J and K
Mata Tila Multipurpose Project	On Betwa in U.P. & M.P.
Thein Project	On Ravi, Punjab
Pong Dam	On Beas, Punjab

Climate of india

Climatic Diversity in the Indian Subcontinent

India has tropical monsoon type of climate. It is greatly influenced by the presence of Himalayas in the North as they block the cold masses from Central Asia.

El Nino and La Nina

El Nino is a narrow warm current, which occasionally appears off the coast of Peru in December by temporarily replacing the cold Peru Current. La Nina is the reverse of El-Nino. It is a harbinger of heavy monsoon showers in India.

Agriculture in India

- About 65–70% of the total population of the country is dependent on agriculture.
- Agriculture with its allied activities accounts for 45% of our national income.

There are three crop seasons in India:

- **Kharif:** Sown in June/July, harvested in September/October, e.g., rice, jowar, bajra, ragi, maize, cotton and jute.
- **Rabi:** Sown in October/December, harvested in April/May, e.g., wheat, barley, peas, rapeseed, mustard grains.
- **Zyad:** They are raised between April/June, e.g., melons, watermelons, cucumbers, *toris*, leafy and other vegetables.

Sources of Irrigation in India

There are various sources of irrigation which are:

(a) **Wells and Tubewells:** 46% of total irrigation.
(b) **Canals:** 39% of total irrigation.
(c) **Tanks:** 8% of total irrigation.
(d) **Other sources:** 7% of total irrigation (Dongs, Kuhls, Springs etc.).

National Highways

- They are constructed and maintained by the Central Government.
- The National Highways has 71,772 km length comprising only 2% of the total length of roads, carries about 40% of the total traffic of India.
- NH7 is the longest National Highway in India.
- NH47 is the shortest highway in the Indian highway network.

State Highways

- They are constructed and maintained by the State Government.
- Maharashtra has the maximum length of roads.

Rail Transport

- The total route covered is approximately 63000 km.
- Indian Railway was nationalised in 1950.
- The management and governance of the Indian Railways is in the hands of the Railway Board.
- Railways have been divided into 17 zones.
- India has the second largest railway network in Asia and the fourth largest in the World after the USA, Russia and China.

Air Transport

- JRD Tata was the first person to take a solo flight from Mumbai to Karachi in 1931.
- In 1935, the 'Tata Airlines' started its operation between Mumbai and Thiruvananthapuram and in 1937 between Mumbai and Delhi.
- Airways in India started in 1911.

Water Transport

- The Central Water Tribunal was established in 1887.
- Its headquarters is in Kolkata.

Internal Waterways

- India has got about 14,544 km of navigable waterways which comprise rivers, canals, backwaters, creeks, etc.
- The Inland Waterways Authority of India (IWAI) came into existence on 27 October, 1986.

Ports in India

- India has about 190 ports, with 13 major and the rest intermediate and minor.
- Largest port of India is Jawaharlal Nehru Port in Mumbai.

Important Indian Towns on Rivers

Town	River
Mathura	Yamuna
Delhi	Yamuna
Agra	Yamuna
Badrinath	Alaknanda
Kanpur	Ganga
Kota	Chambal
Ahmedabad	Sabarmati
Bareilly	Ram Ganga
Ayodhya	Saryu
Lucknow	Gomti
Srinagar	Jhelum
Varanasi	Ganga
Patna	Ganga
Ujjain	Kshipra
Jamshedpur	Swarnarekha
Surat	Tapti
Curnool	Tungabhadra
Vijayvada	Krishna
Nasik	Godavari
Hyderabad	Musi
Tiruchirapalli	Cauvery
Cuttack	Mahanadi
Sambalpur	Mahanadi
Kolkata	Hooghly
Guwahati	Brahmaputra
Dibrugarh	Brahmaputra

Nuclear Power Stations in India

Tarapur	Maharashtra
Kalpakkam	Tamil Nadu, called Indira Gandhi Centre for Atomic Research
Narora	U. P.
Rawatbhata	Kota, Rajasthan
Kaiga	Karnataka
Kakrapar	Gujarat
Kudankulam	Tamil Nadu

Major Thermal Power Plants in India

Neyveli	Tamil Nadu
Korba	Chhattisgarh
Obra	U. P.
Harduaganj	U. P.
Rihand	U. P.
Singrauli	U. P.
Parichha	U. P.
Talcher	Odisha
Farakka	W. Bengal
Satpura	M. P.
Ramagundam	A. P.
Vindhyanchal	M. P.

Exercise

1. **The Paithan (Jayakwadi) Hydro-electric project, completed with the help of Japan, is on the river**
(a) Ganga (b) Cauvery
(c) Narmada (d) Godavari

2. **The percentage of irrigated land in India is about**
(a) 45 (b) 65
(c) 35 (d) 25

3. **The southernmost point of peninsular India, that is, Kanyakumari, is**
(a) north of Tropic of Cancer
(b) south of the Equator
(c) south of the Capricorn
(d) north of the Equator

4. **The pass located at the southern end of the Nilgiri Hills in south India is called**
(a) the Palghat gap
(b) the Bhorghat pass

(c) the Thalgat pass
(d) the Bolan pass

5. Which of the following factors are responsible for the rapid growth of sugar production in south India as compared to north India?
I.Higher per acre field of sugarcane
II.Higher sucrose content of sugarcane
III. Lower labour cost
IV. Longer crushing period
(a) I and II (b) I, II and III
(c) I, III and IV (d) I, II and IV

6. Which of the following rivers does not flow into the Arabian Sea?
(a) Tungabhadra
(b) Sabarmati
(c) Mandovi
(d) Narmada

7. Which of the following is the highest peak of Satpura Range?
(a) Gurushikhar
(b) Dhupgarh
(c) Pachmarhi
(d) Mahendragiri

8. Consider the following Mangrove areas:
1.Bhitarkanika
2.Pichavaram
3.Coondapur
Which among the above is/are situated on the Eastern Coast of India?
(a) Only 1 (b) 1 and 2
(c) 1 and 3 (d) 1, 2 and 3

9. Tropic of Cancer passes through which of the following group of Indian States:
(a) Gujarat, MP, Chhattisgarh, Manipur
(b) Rajasthan, Jharkhand, West Bengal, Mizoram
(c) UP, MP, Bihar, Jharkhand
(d) Maharashtra, Chhattisgarh, Odisha, Andhra Pradesh

10. The land frontier of India is about 15200 KM. Which of the following countries shares the largest border length with India:
(a) Bangladesh (b) Pakistan
(c) China (d) Nepal

11.The lacustrine deposits of Kashmir called 'Karewas' are known for :
(a) Saffron Cultivation
(b) Terrace farming
(c) Apple Orchards
(d) Jhum Cultivation

12. Which of the following Mountain passes forms the 'tri-junction' of India,China and Myanmar?
(a) Nathu La (b) Jelep La
(c) Bomdi La (d) Diphu

13. Which of the following mountain ranges form a dividing line between the Ganges Plain and the Deccan Plateau?
(a) Aravalli (b) Vindhya
(c) Satpura (d) Ajanta

14. The famous hill-station 'Kodaikanal' lies in:
(a) Nilgiri hills
(b) Palani hills
(c) Cardamom hills
(d) Javadi hills

15. The Andaman and Nicobar Islands are submerged parts of mountain range called:
(a) Arakan Yoma
(b)Pegu Yoma
(c) Askai Chin
(d) Tien Shan

16. Which of the following Indian States/UT has the maximum percentage of mangrove cover in the country?
(a) Gujarat
(b) West Bengal
(c) Andaman and Nicobar
(d) Odisha

17. Asia's largest tulip garden is located in which state?
(a) Jammu & Kashmir
(b) Assam
(c) Sikkim
(d) Uttarakhand

18. Barak valley in Assam is famous for which among the following?
(a) Petroleum Production
(b) Tea Cultivation
(c) Bamboo Industry
(d) Cottage Industries

19. Which among the following spreads from Sasaram and Rohtas in Western Bihar to Chittaurgarh in Rajasthan?
(a) Aravali System
(b) Vindhyan System
(c) Dharwar System
(d) Cudappah System

20. The famous "Chatham Saw Mill" is located in which among the following states / union territories of India?
(a) Daman & Diu
(b) Goa
(c) Andaman & Nicobar Islands
(d) Laskhadweep

21. Area wise, which among the following is the largest physiographic unit of India?
(a) Himalayan Mountains
(b) Thar Desert
(c) Deccan Plateau
(d) Great Plains of North India

22. Heritage power project Sonapani mini-hydel power project is located in which state?
(a) Meghalaya
(b) Mizoram
(c) Nagaland
(d) Arunachal Pradesh

23. At which among the following places, Brahamputra takes a U-turn at the time of entering into India?
(a) Kula Kangri
(b) Lunpo Gangri
(c) Namcha Barwa
(d) Noijin Kangsang

24. Jarawas and Sentinelese tribes are found in which among the following state/Union Territory of India?
(a) Andaman & Nicobar Islands
(b) Madhya Pradesh
(c) Lakshadweep
(d) Arunachal Pradesh

25. Tumkur, where Geological Survey of India has found indications of Gold Reserves, is located in which among the following states?
(a) Andhra Pradesh
(b) Karnataka
(c) Tamil nadu
(d) Maharatsra

26. From which of the following countries India does NOT import Uranium?
(a) Kazakhstan (b) Namibia
(c) Brazil (d) Mongolia

27. Which of the following states is/are not a part of Western Ghats?
(a) Gujarat
(b) Tamil Nadu
(c) Andhra Pradesh
(d) Both (b) and (c)

28. The percentage of earth surface covered by India is
(a) 2.4 (b) 3.4
(c) 4.4 (d) 5.4

29. Which among the following is/are the major factor/factors responsible for the monsoon type of climate in India?

I. Location
II. Thermal contrast
III. Upper air circulation
IV. Inter-tropical convergence zone
(a) I
(b) II, III
(c) II, III and IV
(d) I, II, III and IV

30. The present forest area of India, according to satellite data, is
(a) increasing
(b) decreasing
(c) static
(d) decreasing in open forest area but increasing in closed forest area

31. The India's highest annual rainfall is reported at
(a) Namchi, Sikkim
(b) Churu, Rajasthan
(c) Mawsynram, Meghalaya
(d) Chamba, Himachal Pradesh

32. The refineries are Mathura, Digboi and Panipat are set up by
(a) Indian Oil Corporation Ltd.
(b) Hindustan Petroleum Corporation Ltd.
(c) Bharat Petroleum Corporation Ltd.
(d) Crude Distillation unit of Madras Refineries Ltd.

33. The year ____ is called a Great Divide in the demographic history of India.
(a) 1901 (b) 1921
(c) 1941 (d) 1951

34. The only private sector refinery set up by Reliance Petroleum Ltd. is located at
(a) Guwahati (b) Jamnagar
(c) Mumbai (d) Chennai

35. The only state in India that produces saffron is
(a) Assam
(b) Himachal Pradesh
(c) Jammu and Kashmir
(d) Meghalaya

36. Three important rivers of the Indian subcontinent have their sources near the Mansarover Lake in the Great Himalayas. These rivers are
(a) Indus, Jhelum and Sutlej
(b) Brahmaputra, Sutlej and Yamuna
(c) Brahmaputra, Indus and Sutlej
(d) Jhelum, Sutlej and Yamuna

37. The zonal soil type of peninsular India belongs to
(a) red soils (b) yellow soils
(c) black soils (d) older alluvium

38. Which of the following groups of rivers originate from the Himachal mountains?
(a) Beas, Ravi and Chenab
(b) Ravi, Chenab and Jhelum
(c) Sutlej, Beas and Ravi
(d) Sutlej, Ravi and Jhelum

39. Which of the following groups of states has the largest deposits of iron ore?
(a) Andhra Pradesh and Karnataka
(b) Bihar and Orissa
(c) Madhya Pradesh and Maharashtra
(d) West Bengal and Assam

40. Which of the following union territories of India has the highest density of population per sq km?
(a) Pondicherry (b) Lakshadweep
(c) Delhi (d) Chandigarh

41. Which atomic power station in India is built completely indigenously?
(a) Kalpakkam
(b) Narora
(c) Rawat Bhata
(d) Tarapore

42. The south-west monsoon contributes ____ of the total rain in India.
(a) 86% (b) 50%
(c) 22% (d) 100%

43. Which of the following groups of rivers have their source of origin in Tibet?
(a) Brahmaputra, Ganges and Sutlej
(b) Ganges, Sutlej and Yamuna
(c) Brahmaputra, Indus and Sutlej
(d) Chenab, Ravi and Sutlej

44. Which of the following measures are effective for soil conservation in India?
I. Avoiding crop rotation
II. Afforestation
III. Encouraging the use of chemical fertilizers
IV. Limiting shifting cultivation
(a) I and II (b) II and IV
(c) III and IV (d) I, II and III

45. Which of the following crops needs maximum water per hectare?
(a) Barley (b) Maize
(c) Sugarcane (d) Wheat

46. The watershed between India and Myanmar is formed by
(a) the Naga hills
(b) the Garo hills
(c) Khasi hills
(d) the Jaintia hills

47. The originating in the Himalayan mountain complex consists of how many distinct drainage systems of the Indian Subcontinent?
(a) Two (b) Three
(c) Four (d) Five

48. Which of the following crops is regarded as a plantation crop?
(a) Coconut (b) Cotton
(c) Sugarcane (d) Rice

49. Which of the following countries leads in the production of aluminium and its products in the world?
(a) Australia (b) France
(c) India (d) USA

50. The natural region which holds the Indian subcontinent is
(a) equatorial climate change region
(b) hot deset
(c) monsoon
(d) mediterranean

51. The most ideal region for the cultivation of cotton in India is
(a) the Brahmaputra valley
(b) the Indo-Gangetic valley
(c) the Deccan plateau
(d) the Rann of Kutch

52. The number of major ports in India is
(a) 5 (b) 8
(c) 13 (d) 15

53. Which of the following is a peninsular river of India?
(a) Gandak (b) Kosi
(c) Krishna (d) Sutlej

54. Which of the following is the most important raw material for generation of power in India?
(a) Coal
(b) Mineral Oil
(c) Natural Gas
(d) Uranium

55. When it is noon IST at Allahabad in India, the time at Greenwich, London, will be
(a) midnight ,GMT
(b) 1730 hours
(c) 0630 hours
(d) None of the above

56. Which country has the largest coast line?
(a) USA (b) Australia
(c) Canada (d) India

57. The river Godavari is often referred to as Vridha Ganga because
(a) it is the older river of India
(b) of its large size and extent among the peninsular rivers
(c) there are a fairly large number of pilgrimage centres situated on its banks
(d) its length is nearly the same as that of the river Ganges

58. The scarcity or crop failure of which of the following can cause a serious edible oll crisis in India?
(a) coconut (b) Groundnut
(c) Linseed (d) Mustard

59. The pennines (Europe), Appalachians (America) and the Aravallis (India) are examples of
(a) old mountains
(b) young mountains
(c) fold mountains
(d) block mountains

60. The Jhamarkotra mines of Rajasthan are best known for which among the following minerals?
(a) Mica
(b) Zinc
(c) Rock Phosphate
(d) Lime Stone

61. 'Gir Kesar', which has been given the Geographical Indication (GI) tag, is a famous variety of which among the following?
(a) Saffron (b) Pepper
(c) Mango (d) Sweat

62. The Kandaleru Dam is located in which state?
(a) Kerala
(b) Maharashtra
(c) Andhra Pradesh
(d) Goa

63. Pagladia Dam Project is located in which state?
(a) Arunachal Pradesh
(b) Sikkim
(c) Assam
(d) West Bengal

64. Prior to Census 2011, in which among the following census highest Sex Ratio was recorded in India?
(a) Census 1941
(b) Census 1951
(c) Census 1961
(d) Census 1971

65. Which among the following rivers is known as Yarlung Tsangpo in Tibet?
(a) Indus (b) Yamuna
(c) Ganges (d) Brahamputra

66. Which among the following was steel plant of India is sometimes called India's First Swadeshi Steel Plant?
(a) Bengal Iron Works Company
(b) TISCO
(c) IISCO
(d) Bokaro Steel Plant

67. In which of the following states, India's maximum number of mines producing minerals (excluding minor minerals, petroleum (crude), natural gas and atomic minerals) are located?
(a) Gujarat
(b) Andhra Pradesh
(c) Jharkhand
(d) Madhya Pradesh

68. Which among the following coal producer of India is outside the Coal India Ltd?
(a) Southern Eastern Coalfields (Bilaspur)
(b) Bharat Coking Coal (Dhanbad)
(c) Mahanandi Coalfields (Sambalpur)
(d) Singerani Collieries Company (Telangana)

69. An Inland water transit and trade protocol exists between India and which among the following neighbors?
(a) Sri Lanka (b) Bangladesh
(c) Pakistan (d) Myanmar

70. Which among the following is the largest district of Maharashtra in terms of Area?
(a) Aurangabad
(b) Ahamednagar
(c) Sindhudurg
(d) Latur

71. Which among the following is not a member country of the Mekong Ganga Cooperation?
(a) India
(b) Bangladesh
(c) Thailand
(d) Vietnam

72. Which among the following is a geology award given annually by Indian Geophysical Union?
(a) Dr. BC Roy Award
(b) Siva Prasad Barooah National Award
(c) M. S. Krishanan Award
(d) Karmaveer Puraskaar

73. Which among the following is the only place in India, where Chinese Fishing Nets are used outside China?
(a) Pondicherry
(b) Kochi
(c) Kolkata
(d) Bhubneshwar

74. Saddam Beach is located in which state?
(a) Tamil Nadu
(b) Kerala
(c) Maharastra
(d) Karnataka

75. Which of the following variety of Marble is found in India?
(a) Makrana
(b) Bhainslana
(c) Phrygia
(d) Carrara

76. In which year , Dakshin Gangotri, India's first settlement in Antarctica got buried in Ice?
(a) 1980 (b) 1985
(c) 1987 (d) 1989

77. Temi Tea Garden is located in which state?
(a) Meghalaya (b) Sikkim
(c) Assam
(d) West Bengal

78. Damodar and Sone river valley and Rajmahal hills in the eastern India are depository of the______.
(a) Cuddappa System Rocks
(b) Dharwar System Rocks
(c) Gondwana System Rocks
(d) Vindhyan System Rocks

79. Port Pipavav, which is the first private sector port in India, is located in which of the following states?
(a) West Bengal
(b) Maharashtra
(c) Gujarat
(d) Andhra Pradesh

80. Which among the following boards is defunct now?
(a) Tea Board of India
(b) Rubber Board
(c) National Biotechnology Board
(d) None of them

81. Which among the following is the latest refinery established?
(a) Digboi (b) Panipat
(c) Trombay (d) Vishakapatnam

82. "Ambassa" was in news as the Geological Survey of India has found huge reserves of coal. In which state Ambasa is located?
(a) Meghalaya (b) Tripura
(c) Assam (d) Nagaland

83. Which among the following is sometimes known as "Third Pole"?
(a) Hudson Highlands
(b) Rocky Mountains
(c) Severny Island ice cap
(d) Siachen Glacier

84. Indian Institute of Crop Processing Technology is located in?
(a) Madurai (b) Thanjaur
(c) Kochi (d) Ooty

85. Which of the following city of Tamil Nadu is known as world's largest producer and most important trading center of turmeric in Asia?
(a) Athoor (b) Karaikudi
(c) Thanjavur (d) Erode

86. Multi-modal International Cargo Hub and Airport (MIHAN) project is in which of the following cities?
(a) Mangalore (b) Hyderabad
(c) Pune (d) Nagpur

87. Which of the following states has largest coastline?
(a) Gujarat
(b) Andhra Pradesh
(c) Maharastra
(d) Tamilnadu

88. Which among the following part of Bombay (now Mumbai) is known as Old Woman's Island?
(a) Parel (b) Worli
(c) Colaba (d) Mazgaon

89. The Jakham Dam is located in which state?
(a) Madhya Pradesh
(b) Gujarat
(c) Rajasthan
(d) Uttar Pradesh

90. Which among the following group of states represents one third of India's cattle population?
(a) Uttar Pradesh, Bihar, Maharastra
(b) Punjab, Orissa, Rajasthan
(c) Karnataka, Rajasthan, Andhra Pradesh
(d) Madhya Pradesh, West Bengal,Uttar Pradesh

91. Which among the following tribe has the largest population in India?
(a) Bhils (b) Meenas
(c) Gonds (d) Sahariyas

92. Bring out the inly mentioned location:
(a) Pasteur Institute of India: Coonoor
(b) National TB Training Institute - Bangalore
(c) Central leprosy Training & Research institute - Chengalpattu
(d) Kasturba Health Society - Ahamadabad

93. Which among the following is sometimes known as "Third Pole"?
(a) Hudson Highlands
(b) Rocky Mountains
(c) Severny Island ice cap
(d) Siachen Glacier

94. "Ambassa" was in news as the Geological Survey of India has found huge reserves of coal. In which state Ambasa is located?
(a) Meghalaya (b) Tripura
(c) Assam (d) Nagaland

95. Which among the following is not matched correctly:
(a) Steel Authority of India Ltd (SAIL) : New Delhi
(b) MECON Ltd. : Ranchi
(c) Hindustan Steel Works Construction Ltd (HSCL) : Kolkata
(d) Ferro Scrap Nigam Ltd.(FSNL) : Bokaro

96. Which among the following is the latest refinery established?
(a) Digboi (b) Panipat
(c) Trombay (d) Vishakapatnam

Answers

1. (d)	**2.** (c)	**3.** (d)	**4.** (a)	**5.** (d)	**6.** (a)	**7.** (b)	**8.** (b)	**9.** (b)	**10.** (a)
11. (a)	**12.** (d)	**13.** (b)	**14.** (b)	**15.** (a)	**16.** (b)	**17.** (a)	**18.** (b)	**19.** (b)	**20.** (c)
21. (c)	**22.** (a)	**23.** (c)	**24.** (a)	**25.** (b)	**26.** (c)	**27.** (c)	**28.** (a)	**29.** (d)	**30.** (b)
31. (c)	**32.** (a)	**33.** (b)	**34.** (b)	**35.** (c)	**36.** (c)	**37.** (a)	**38.** (a)	**39.** (b)	**40.** (c)
41. (a)	**42.** (a)	**43.** (c)	**44.** (b)	**45.** (c)	**46.** (a)	**47.** (b)	**48.** (a)	**49.** (d)	**50.** (c)
51. (c)	**52.** (c)	**53.** (c)	**54.** (a)	**55.** (c)	**56.** (c)	**57.** (b)	**58.** (b)	**59.** (a)	**60.** (c)
61. (c)	**62.** (c)	**63.** (c)	**64.** (c)	**65.** (d)	**66.** (d)	**67.** (b)	**68.** (d)	**69.** (b)	**70.** (b)
71. (b)	**72.** (c)	**73.** (b)	**74.** (b)	**75.** (a)	**76.** (d)	**77.** (b)	**78.** (c)	**79.** (c)	**80.** (c)
81. (b)	**82.** (b)	**83.** (d)	**84.** (b)	**85.** (d)	**86.** (d)	**87.** (a)	**88.** (c)	**89.** (c)	**90.** (d)
91. (a)	**92.** (d)	**93.** (d)	**94.** (b)	**95.** (d)	**96.** (b)				

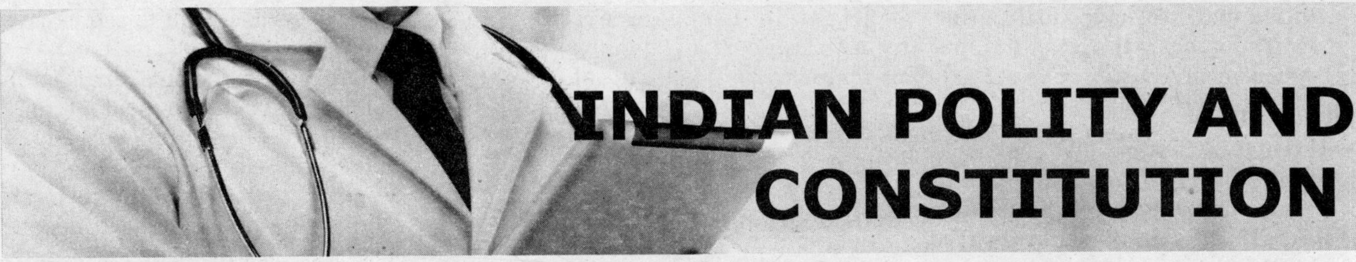

Constitution

Constitution is the foundational law of a country which ordains the fundamental principles on which the government (or the governance) of that country is based. With the exception of the United Kingdom, almost all democratic countries possess a written constitution.

Evolution of Indian Constitution

The first Constitution of India framed and given to themselves by the people of India was adopted by the Constituent Assembly on 26 November 1949. It came into full effect from 26 January 1950. The Constitution as originally adopted had 22 parts, 395 articles and 8 schedules.

Constituent Assembly and Making of the Constitution

- The Cabinet Mission envisaged the establishment of a Constituent Assembly to frame a Constitution for the country. Members of the Constituent Assembly were elected by the Provincial Legislative Assemblies.
- After the partition of India, number of members of the Constituent Assembly came to 299, of whom 284 were actually present on 26 November 1949 and signed on the finally approved Constitution of India Assembly, which had been elected for undivided India, held its first meeting on December 9, 1946, and reassembled on August 14, 1947, as the sovereign Constituent Assembly for the dominion of India.
- It took **two years, eleven months and eighteen days** for the Constituent Assembly to finalise the Constitution.
- The Assembly appointed the Drafting Committee with Dr. B.R. Ambedkar as the Chairman on August 29, 1947.
- The members of the Drafting Committee were N. Gopalaswamy Ayyangar, Alladi Krishnaswamy Ayya, K.M. Munshi, Mohd. Saadullah, B.L. Mitter (later replaced by N. Madhava Rao), and Dr. D.P. Khaitan (replaced on death by T.T. Krishnamachari).
- **Dr. Sachidanand Sinha** was the first President of the Constituent Assembly
- **Dr. Rajendra Prasad** was elected as the President of the Assembly.

Enactment of the Constitution

On November 26, 1949, Constitution was adopted, containing Preamble and 395 Articles, 18 Parts and 8 Schedules. The Constitution in its current form consists of a Preamble, 24 Parts, 448 Articles and 12 Schedules.

Enforcement of the Constitution

The Constitution came into force on January 26, 1950.

Salient features of the constitution

- Parliamentary Government
- India has a parliamentary system of government both at the centre and at the states. The president is the head of the union of India and the Governors are head of the states but they act on the advice of the council of ministers. They have nominal powers.
- **Federal system with unitary features:** Our constitution contains federal features of government like division of powers written constitution, independent judiciary and bicameralism but a large number of unitary features like a strong center, single citizenship flexibility of constitution, integrated judiciary emergency provisions etc.
- Independent Judiciary
- Secular state
- Emergency provisions

Schedules of the Indian Constitution

1st Schedule: 29 States and 7 Union Territories with Territorial demarcations.

2nd Schedule: Part 'A' Salary and emoluments of the President and Governors of States.

Part 'B' Omitted.

Part 'C' Salary and emoluments of the Speaker/Deputy Speaker or Chairman/Vice-Chairman of the Lok Sabha, Rajya Sabha and State Legislative Assemblies or Councils.

Part 'D' Salary and emoluments of the judge of the Supreme Court and High Courts.

Part 'E' Salary and emoluments of the Comptroller and Auditor General of India.

3rd Schedule: Forms of oath and affirmations of members of legislatures, ministers and judges.

4th Schedule: Allocation of seats to States and Union Territories in the Rajya Sabha.

5th Schedule: Administration and control of Scheduled Areas and STs.

6th Schedule: Administration of Tribal Areas of North-Eastern States.

7th Schedule: Distribution of power between the Union and the State Government. (Union List, State List and Concurrent List).

8th Schedule: Description of 22 languages recognised by the constitution.

9th Schedule: Validation of certain Acts and Regulations.

10th Schedule: Provisions as to disqualification on ground of defection (Anti-defection Law introduced by the 52nd Constitutional Amendment Act).

11th Schedule: Power, authority and responsibilities of Panchayats, 29 subjects over which the Panchayats have jurisdiction (refer to the 73rd Constitutional Amendment Act).

12th Schedule: Powers, authority and responsibilities of Municipalities, 18 subjects over which the

Municipalities have jurisdiction (refer to the 74th Constitutional Amendment Act).

The Preamble

- **Text of the Preamble:** "We, the People of India having solemnly resolved to constitute India into a **Sovereign Socialist Secular Democratic Republic** and to secure to all citizens **Justice**, social, economic and political; **Liberty** of thought, expression, belief, faith and worship, **Equality** of status and of opportunity; and to promote among them all **Fraternity** assuring the dignity of the individual and the unity and integrity of the Nation in our Constituent Assembly on this twenty-sixth day of November, 1949, do hereby adopt, enact and give to ourselves this constitution."
- The Preamble to the Indian Constitution is based on the **Objectives Resolution** drafted and moved by Pandit Nehru and adopted by the Constituent Assembly.
- The Preamble is **not enforceable in a court of law**.
- The Preamble has been amended only once so far, in 1976, by 42nd Constitutional Amendment Act, which added three new words **Socialist, Secular** and **Integrity.** This amendment was held to be valid.

Fundamental Rights

- The Fundamental Rights have been described in **Articles 12-35**, Part III of Indian Constitution.
- Right to Freedom articles 19-22.
- Right against Exploitation Articles 23-24
- Right to Freedom of religion Articles 25-28
- Cultural and Educational Rights Articles 29-30
- Right to Constitutional Remedies Article-32
- The Writs
- Right to Information

Fundamental Duties

In 1976, the FDs of citizens were added by 42nd **Constitutional Amendment Act** on the basis of Swaran Singh Committee Report.

List of Fundamental Duties

According to **Article 51A**, it shall be the duty of every citizen of India:

- To abide by the Constitution and respect its ideals and institutions, the National Flag and the National Anthem;
- To cherish and follow the noble ideals that inspired the national struggle for freedom;
- To uphold and protect the sovereignty, unity and integrity of India;
- To promote harmony and the spirit of common brotherhood amongst all the people of India transcending religious, linguistic and regional or sectional diversities and to renounce practices derogatory to the dignity of women;
- To defend the country and render national service, when called upon to do so;
- To value and preserve the rich heritage of the country's composite culture;
- To protect and improve the natural environment including forests, lakes, rivers and wildlife and to have compassion for living creatures;
- To develop scientific temper, humanism and the spirit of inquiry and reform;
- To safeguard public property and to abjure violence;
- To strive toward excellence in all spheres of individual and collective activity so that the nation constantly rises to higher levels of endeavour and achievement; and
- To provide opportunities for education to his child or ward between the age of 6 to 14 years. This duty was added by the 86th Constitutional Amendment Act, 2002.

Executive of the Union

The President

- President is the head of the Union Executive.
- The President of India is indirectly elected by an electoral college, in accordance with the system of proportional representation by means of the single transferable vote.
- The Electoral College for the president consists of:
  - The elected members of both Houses of Parliament;
  - The elected members of the Legislative Assemblies of the states; and
  - The elected members of the Legislative Assemblies of Union Territories of Delhi and Pondicherry (now Puducherry).

Term of the President

Under Article 56, the President shall hold office for a term of five year from the date on which he enters upon his office.

Presidents of India

S.No.	Name	Period
1.	Rajendra Prasad	26 Jan. 1950 to 13 May 1962
2.	Sarvapalli Radhakrishnan	13 May 1962 to 13 May 1967
3.	Zakir Hussain	13 May 1967 to 3 May 1969
4.	Varahagiri Venkata Giri	3 May 1969 to 20 July 1969
5.	Muhammad Hidayatullah	20 July 1969 to 24 Aug. 1969
6.	Varahagiri Venkata Giri	24 Aug. 1969 to 24 Aug. 1974
7.	Fakhruddin Ali Ahmed	24 Aug. 1974 to 11 Feb. 1977
8.	Basappa Danappa Jatti	11 Feb. 1977 to 25 July 1977
9.	Neelam Sanjiva Reddy	25 July 1977 to 25 July 1982
10.	Giani Zail Singh	25 July 1982 to 25 July 1987
11.	Ramaswamy Venkataraman	25 July 1987 to 25 July 1992
12.	Shankar Dayal Sharma	25 July 1992 to 25 July 1997

13.	Kocheril Raman Narayanan	25 July 1997 to 25 July 2002
14.	A.P.J. Abdul Kalam	25 July 2002 to 25 July 2007
15.	Pratibha Patil	25 July 2007 to 25 July 2012
16.	Pranab Mukherjee	25 July 2012 to 25 July 2017
17.	Ramnath Kobind	25 July 2017 to till date

The Vice-President

- Vice-President is indirectly elected by means of single transferable vote.
- State Legislatures do not take part in the election of Vice-President.
- Electoral College of Vice-President consists of elected and nominated members of both the Houses of Parliament.
- All disputes regarding election of Vice-President are adjudicated by the Supreme Court.

Term of Office Under Article 67

- Holds office for a **term of 5 years** from the date on which he enters upon his office.
- Can be removed by a resolution of the Rajya Sabha passed by an absolute majority and agreed by the Lok Sabha [Article 67 (b)].

The Prime Minister and the Union Council of Ministers

Prime Minister

Prime Minister is the head of the government while President is the head of the State of the Republic of India. **Article 75 says** that the Prime Minister shall be appointed by the President.

Oath, Term and Salary

The **term of the Prime Minister is not fixed** and he holds office during the pleasure of the President. However, this does not mean that the President can dismiss the Prime Minister at any time. So long as the Prime Minister enjoys the majority support in the Lok Sabha, he cannot be dismissed by the President. However, if he loses the confidence of the Lok Sabha, he must resign or the President can dismiss him.

Prime Ministers of India

S.No.	Name	Period
1.	Jawahar Lal Nehru	15 Aug. 1947 to 27 May 1964
2.	Gulzarilal Nanda	27 May 1964 to 9 June 1964
3.	Lal Bahadur Shastri	09 June 1964 to 11 Jan. 1966
4.	Gulzarilal Nanda	11 Jan. 1966 to 24 Jan. 1966
5.	Indira Gandhi	24 Jan. 1966 to 24 March 1977
6.	Morarji Desai	24 March 1977 to 28 July 1979
7.	Charan Singh	28 July 1979 to 14 Jan. 1980
8.	Indira Gandhi	14 Jan. 1980 to 31 Oct. 1984
9.	Rajiv Gandhi	31 Oct. 1984 to 2 Dec. 1989
10.	Vishwanath Pratap Singh	2 Dec.1989 to 10 Nov. 1990
11.	Chandra Shekhar	10 Nov 1990 to 21 June 1991
12.	P.V. Narasimha Rao	21 June 1991 to 16 May 1996
13.	Atal Behari Vajpayee	16 May 1996 to 1 June 1996
14.	H.D. Deve Gowda	1 June 1996 to 21 April 1997
15.	Atal Behari Vajpayee	19 March 1998 to 22 May 2004
16.	Dr. Manmohan Singh	22 May 2004 to 26 May 2014
17.	Narendra Modi	26 May 2014 to till date

Appointment of Ministers

Ministers are appointed by the President on the advice of the Prime Minister.

Oath and Salary of Ministers

President administers the oath to the Ministers.

Responsibility of Ministers

Under Article 75, the CoMs is collectively responsible to Lok Sabha for all their acts.

Deputy Prime Minister

The post of Deputy Prime Minister is not mentioned in the Constitution.

List of Deputy Prime Ministers

Name	Tenure
Sardar Vallabhbhai Patel	1947–1950
Morarji Desai	1967–1969
Charan Singh and Jagjiven Ram	1979–1979
Y. B. Chavan	1979–1980
Devi Lal	1989–1990
Devi Lal	1990–1991
L. K. Advani	2002–2004

The Attorney General of India

- The Attorney General is the first Law Officer of the Government of India.

- The Attorney General for India is appointed by the President and holds office during the pleasure of the President. He must have the same qualifications as required to be a Judge of the Supreme Court.
- The Attorney General for India is not a member of the Cabinet. But he has the right to speak in the Houses of Parliament or in any Committee thereof, but he has no right to vote.
- He is entitled to the privileges of a Member of Parliament. In the performance of his official duties, the Attorney General has the right of audience in all Courts in the territory of India.

The Comptroller and Auditor General of India

- Though appointed by the President, the Comptroller and Auditor General can be grounded of proved misbehaviour or incapacity.
- His salary and conditions of service are laid down by Parliament and cannot be varied to his disadvantage during his term of office.
- The term of office of the Comptroller and Auditor General (CAG) is 6 years from the date on which he assumes office.
- CAG vacates office on attaining the age of 65 years even without completing the 6-year term. He can resign by writing under his hand, addressed to the President of India.
- His salary is equal to that of a Judge of the Supreme Court.

The Parliament of India

- The Parliament of India consists of the President, the Lok Sabha and the Rajya Sabha (Article 79).
- Out of seven UTs only two (Delhi and Puducherry) have representation in the Rajya Sabha.

Rajya Sabha [Article 80]

- Rajya Sabha is a permanent body and **not subject to dissolution.** Its maximum strength is 250. The total membership of the present Rajya Sabha is 245 however one-third members retire every second year. Their seats are filled up by fresh elections and presidential nomination at the beginning of every third year.
- There are no seats reserved for SCs and STs in Rajya Sabha.
- Representation of People Act (1951) provided the term of office of a member of the Rajya Sabha shall be **six years.**

Lok Sabha [Article 81]

- Its maximum strength is 550 + 2 members of its Anglo-Indian Community, which includes 530 members from States and 20 from Union Territories. Present strength of Lok Sabha is 545.
- The representatives of the States are directly elected by the people of the States on the basis of adult suffrage.
- Every citizen who is not less than 18 years of age and is not otherwise disqualified is entitled to vote at such election.
- The normal term of the Lok Sabha is 5 years, but it may be dissolved earlier by the President.
- The normal term of Lok Sabha can be extended by an Act passed by Parliament itself during Emergency.
- The extension cannot be made for a period exceeding one year at a time.
- Such extension cannot continue beyond a period of six months after the proclamation of Emergency ceases to operate.
- Parliament must meet at least twice a year and not more than six months shall elapse between two sessions of Parliament.

Speaker and Deputy Speaker of The Lok Sabha

- He is elected by Lok Sabha from amongst its members, as soon as, after the first meeting.
- He remains in his office during the life of the Lok Sabha. He vacates office earlier in any of the following cases:
- If he ceases to be member of Lok Sabha;
- If he resigns by writing to the Deputy Speaker; and
- If he is removed by a resolution passed by a majority of all the members of the Lok Sabha. Such a resolution can be moved only after giving 14 days advance notice.

Deputy Speaker

Anthasayanam Ayyangar was the First Deputy Speaker of Lok Sabha.

Special Power of Rajya Sabha

Due to its federal character, the Rajya Sabha has been given two exclusive or special powers that are not enjoyed by the Lok Sabha.

1. It can authorise the Parliament to make a law on a subject enumerated in the State List (Article 249).
2. It can authorise the Parliament to create new all-India Service (Common for both the Centre and States (Article 312).

Chairman and Deputy Chairman of the Rajya Sabha

- Vice-President of India is ex-officio Chairman of the Rajya Sabha and functions as the Presiding Officer of that House so long as he does not officiate as the President.
- The Chairman may be removed from his office only if he is **removed** from the office of the Vice-President.

Executive of the States: the Governor

- The Governor is the Constitutional Head of the State and the same Governor can act as Governor of more than one State (Articles 153 and 154).
- Under **Article 155,** the Governor is appointed by the President. **Article 156** states that the Governor holds office during the pleasure of the President.

Tenure of Governor Under Article 156

(a) The Governor shall hold office during the pleasure of the President;
(b) He may resign by writing under the hand addressed to the President;
(c) He holds office for a period of 5 years.
(d) There is no bar to a person being appointed Governor more than once.

Chief Minister's (CM) Appointment

Article 164, says that Chief Minister shall be appointed by the Governor of the State.

Oath, Term and Salary

- Oath of the office of Chief Minister is administered by the Governor to person appointed for this purpose.

- A person, who is not a member of State Legislature can be appointed but he has to get himself elected within 6 months otherwise he is removed.
- The **term of the CM is not fixed** and he holds office during the pleasure of the Governor.
- He cannot be dismissed by the Governor as long as he enjoys the majority support in the Legislative Assembly. But, if he loses the confidence of the Assembly, he must resign or the Governor can dismiss him.

The Supreme Court

- **Article 124** states the establishment and constitution of Supreme Court.
- Every Judge of the Supreme Court, after consulting the Chief Justice of the Supreme Court, is appointed by the President of India.
- At present, the Supreme Court consists of 31 Judges (one CJI and 30 Judges).

Tenure of Judges

The Constitution makes the following provisions:

- Holds office **until he attains the age of 65 years**.
- Resign his office by writing to the President.
- Removed from his office by the President on the recommendation of the Parliament.

Constitutional Bench

A bench consisting of at least 5 judges constituted by the CJI to hear a case involving a substantial question of law.

The High Court

- Accordingly, the President determines the strength of a High Court from time-to-time depending upon its workload.
- The territorial jurisdiction of a High Court is co-terminus with the territory of a State.

Finance Commission

- The Constitution provides for the establishment of a Finance Commission (Articles 272, 273, 275, and 280) by the President.
- The Finance Commission consists of a Chairman and four other members.
- According to the qualifications prescribed by the Parliament, the Chairman is selected among persons who have had experience in public affairs.
- The Commission submits its recommendations to the President which are generally accepted by the Central Government. The recommendations of the Commission are applicable for a period of five years.

Public Service Commissions

- A Joint Public Service Commission can be created by Parliament in pursuance of a resolution passed by the State Legislatures concerned.
- The Union Public Service Commission can serve the needs of a State, if so requested by the Governor of that State and approved by the President.
- Appointment, determination of number of members of the Commission and their conditions of service is done by:
  - The President in the case of the Union or a Joint Commission, and
  - The Governor of State in the case of a State Commission.
- Half of the members of Commission should be persons who have held office under the Government of India or of a State for at least 10 years (Article 316).
- The term of service of a member of a Commission is 6 years from the date of his entering upon office, or until the age of retirement, whichever is earlier.
- Age of retirement for a member of UPSC is **65 years**.
- Age of retirement for a member of PSC of a State or a Joint Commission is **62 years**.
- Services of a member of a Public Service Commission can be terminated by:
  - Resignation in writing addressed to the President (to the Governor in the case of a State Commission).
  - Removal by the President.
- The expenses of the Commission are charged on the Consolidated Fund of India or of the Sate (as the case may be).
- The Chairman of the UPSC is ineligible for further employment either under the Government of India or under the Government of a State.
- The Chairman of a State Public Service Commission is eligible for appointment as the Chairman or member of the Union Public Service Commission or as the Chairman of any other State Public Service Commission, but not for any other employment either under the Government of India or under the Government of a State.
- A member of a State Public Service Commission is eligible for appointment as the Chairman of a State Public Service Commission and Chairman or member of UPSC, but not for any other employment either under the Government of India or under the Government of a State.

Election Commission

- The Election Commission was established in accordance with the Constitution on 25 January 1950.
- The Election Commission consists of a Chief Election Commissioner and two other Election Commissioners.
- President can determine the number of Election Commissioners.

Chief Election Commissioner (CEC)

- The President appoints the Chief Election Commissioner, who has tenure of 6 years, or up to the age of 65 years, whichever is earlier.
- The CEC enjoys the same status and receives the same salary and perks as available to Judges of the Supreme Court.
- The Chief Election Commissioner can be removed from his office only in a manner and on the grounds prescribed for removal of Judge of the Supreme Court.
- Other Election Commissioners can be removed by the President on the recommendation of the Chief Election Commissioner.

Exercise

1. **The minimum age for being eligible to become the Prime Minister of India is**
(a) 21 years (b) 25 years
(c) 30 years (d) 35 years
2. **Which one of the following is not mentioned in the Indian constitution?**
(a) Election Commission
(b) Planning Co: mission
(c) Public Service Commission
(d) Finance Commission
3. **When was the constituent assembly established to frame the constitution of India?**
(a) 10th June, 1946
(b) 6th December, 1946
(c) 26th November, 1949
(d) 26th December,1949
4. **The number of articles in the Indian constitution at the time of its ad was**
(a) 350 (b) 360
(c) 390 (d) 395
5. **When was the President's succession act enacted?**
(a) 1955 (b) 1959
(c) 1964 (d) 1969
6. **In a parliamentary system, the executive is responsible to**
(a) the legislature
(b) the judiciary
(c) the people
(d) none of these
7. **Who enjoys the right to impose reasonable restrictions on the Fundamental Rights?**
(a) The President
(b) The Supreme Court
(c) The Parliament
(d) The Lok Sabha
8. **How many times the President has declared the financial emergency?**
(a) once (b) twice
(c) thrice (d) never
9. **Who decides the disputes regarding the election of the President?**
(a) The Speaker
(b) The Supreme Court
(c) The Election Commission
(d) The Parliament
10. **How many seats are reserved for Union Territories in the Lok Sabha?**
(a) 10 seats (b) 15 seats
(c) 20 seats (d) 30 seats
11. **Who is legally competent to declare war?**
(a) The President
(b) The Prime Minister
(c) The Lok Sabha
(d) The Parliament
12. **Fundamental duties were introduced in the Indian constitution by the**
(a) 40th Amendment
(b) 42nd Amendment
(c) 43rd Amendment
(d) 44th Amendment
13. **Directive principles of state policy are directly concerned with**
(a) Fundamental rights
(b) Fundamental duties
(c) Gandhian principles
(d) Preamble
14. **What is the Maximum age prescribed for election as President of India?**
(a) 58 years (b) 60 years
(c) 62 years (d) no such limit
15. **The President of India can declare emergency**
(a) on his own
(b) on the recommendations of the council of Ministers
(c) on the recommendations of the Prime Minister
(d) on the recommendations of the Parliament
16. **The preamble to the Indian constitution was amended by the**
(a) 24th Amendment
(b) 36th Amendment
(c) 42nd Amendment
(d) 44th Amendment
17. **Who is the chairman of the thirteenth finance commission of India?**
(a) K.C. Pant
(b) Y.B. Chawan
(c) A. M.Khusro
(d) Vijay Kelkar
18. **Who has the right to convince the joint session of the two houses of Parliament in India?**
(a) The Prime Minister
(b) The President
(c) The Vice-President
(d) None of them
19. **The Chief source of political power in India is**
(a) the people
(b) the constitution
(c) the parliament
(d) the parliament and the state legislatures
20. **The Prime Minister is the**
(a) Head of the State
(b) Head of the Government
(c) Head of the State and the head of the Government
(d) None of these
21. **Under which High Court Andaman & Nicobar Islands come?**
(a) Madras High Court
(b) Kerala High Court
(c) Andhra Pradesh High Court
(d) Calcutta High Court
22. **Which article accords special status to Jammu & Kashmir?**
(a) 356 (b) 360
(c) 372 (d) 370
23. **The union territories of India are administered by the**
(a) President
(b) Prime Minister
(c) Defence Minister
(d) Chief Minister
24. **Untouchability comes under which fundamental rights in the Indian constitution?**
(a) Right to freedom
(b) Right to equality
(c) Right against exploitation
(d) Right to freedom of religion
25. **Organisation of village panchayats are in corporated under which head in the Indian constitution?**
(a) Fundamental rights
(b) Citizenship
(c) Directive principles of the state
(d) Fundamental duties
26. **The Chief Justice of the Supreme Court is appointed by**
(a) The President
(b) The Prime Minister
(c) The Parliament
(d) The Law Minister
27. **Who will act as the President of India when the offices of both the President and the Vice-President are vacant?**
(a) The Chief Election Commissioner
(b) The Prime Minister

(c) The Chief Justice of India
(d) The Speaker of Lok Sabha

28. Who has the right to convene the joint session of the two houses of parliament in India?
(a) The Prime Minister
(b) The President
(c) The Vice-President
(d) None of them

29. The planning commission was created in
(a) 1950 A.D (b) 1952 A.D
(c) 1953 A.D (d) 1954 A.D

30. The first citizen of India is the
(a) President
(b) Vice-President
(c) Prime Minister
(d) Speaker

31. The emergency provisions of Indians constitution were borrowed from
(a) Government of India Act, 1935
(b) Soviet Union
(c) Constitution of USA
(d) Weimer constitution of Germany

32. After great labour, the constitution was ready on
(a) 26th December, 1949
(b) 26th January, 1950
(c) 26th November, 1949
(d) 30th November, 1949

33. Indian constitution is often called
(a) Lawyer's paradise
(b) Dictatorial constitution
(c) Evolved constitution
(d) Enacted constitution

34. At present the right to property is merely a
(a) legal right (b) moral right
(c) natural right (d) none of these

35. The term of the office of the President is
(a) 2 years (b) 4 years
(c) 6 years (d) 5 years

36. Lower house of the Indian Parliament is known as
(a) Lok Sabha (b) Rajya Sabha
(c) Assembly (d) Council

37. The highest appeal court in a state is
(a) Session court
(b) Supreme court
(c) Magistrate court
(d) High court

38. Who was the permanent chairman of the constituent assembly?
(a) Dr.Rajendra Prasad
(b) Dr.Ambedkar
(c) Pandit Jawaharlal Nehru
(d) Mahatma Gandhi

39. Freedom of religion is included in articles?
(a) 25-27 (b) 25-28
(c) 26-29 (d) 24-27

40. Which one of the following statements is not correct?
(a) Equal representation is given to states in Rajya Sabha
(b) The Central Government is very strong
(c) Both the Center and the States can legislate on concurrent list
(d) Residuary powers are with the centre

41. Indian upper house is known as
(a) the house of people
(b) the council of states
(c) parliament
(d) none of these

42. The first civil service commission in India was set up on the basis of recommendation of
(a) Aichison Commission
(b) Lee Commission
(c) Simon Commission
(d) Planning Commission

43. The constitution provides for the setting up of the Finance Commission every
(a) year (b) third year
(c) fifth year (d) seventh year

44. The constitution of India was adopted by the
(a) Constituent Assembly
(b) First Parliament
(c) Lok Sabha
(d) Drafting Committee

45. Normally the Parliament can legislate on the subjects enumerated in
(a) the union list
(b) the concurrent list
(c) the state list
(d) the union as well as the concurrent list

46. The constitution of India vests the executive authority of the union in the
(a) President
(b) Council of Ministers
(c) President and Parliament
(d) Prime Minister

47. According to the constitution the upper house of the state legislative can be created or abolished by
(a) The State Legislative Assembly
(b) The Parliament of India
(c) The Governor of the State
(d) Presidential order

48. Which state legislative assembly has the maximum strength?
(a) Andhra Pradesh
(b) West Bengal
(c) Uttar Pradesh
(d) Maharashtra

49. Which one of the following categories of members are not included in the legislative council?
(a) Members elected by Municipalities, District Boards and other local authorities in the state.
(b) Representatives of temple, churches and mosques.
(c) Representatives of persons engaged in teaching in institutions not lower in standard than secondary school
(d) Members nominated by the Governor from amongst persons having special knowledge of literature, science, art, cooperative movements and social service

50. Who had played key role in the formation of Lokpal Bill in India?
(a) Baba Amte
(b) Anna Hajare
(c) Vipin Hazarika
(d) Kiran Bedi

51. The Residuary powers of legislation under Indian Constitution rests with
(a) President (b) Prime Minister
(c) Parliament (d) States

52. Appointments for all India Services are made by
(a) UPSC
(b) President
(c) Prime Minister
(d) Parliament

53. Right to Constitutional Remedies comes under ________.
(a) Legal rights
(b) Fundamental rights
(c) Human rights
(d) Natural rights

54. he Comptroller and Auditor-General of India submits his report relating to the accounts of the Union to the ________.
(a) Finance Minister
(b) Prime Minister

(c) President
(d) Chief Justice of the Supreme Court

55. In a Parliamentary form of Government ________.
(a) The Legislature is responsible to the Judiciary
(b) The Executive is responsible to the Legislature.
(c) The Legislature is responsible to the Executive
(d) The Judiciary is responsible to the Legislature

56. Which of the following statements is correct about the President of India ?
(a) Addresses first session of Parliament after each General Election.
(b) Addresses first session of Parliament at the beginning of each year
(c) Addresses every session of Parliament
(d) Never addresses Parliament

57. Right to Privacy comes under ____.
(a) Article 19 (b) Article 20
(c) Article 21 (d) Article 18

58. What is the meaning of "Public Interest Litigation"?
(a) Anything of public interest
(b) A case brought by victim to court, involving public interest.
(c) A case brought by anyone to court involving public interest.
(d) A directive issued by Supreme Court involving public interest

59. Who appoints and dismisses the gazetted officials of the Union Government?
(a) The President of India
(b) The Prime Minister of India
(c) The Home Minister of India
(d) The Finance Minister of India

60. Which of the following is a name of US Parliament?
(a) Diet
(b) Senate
(c) Congress
(d) House of Commons

61. Which of the following is not provided in the constitution ?
(a) Election Commission
(b) Finance Commission
(c) Public Service Commission
(d) Planning Commission

62. The Comptroller and Auditor General of India does not audit the receipts and expenditure of
(a) Central Government
(b) Local Bodies
(c) State Government
(d) Government Companies

63. The minimum number of members that must be present to hold the meeting of the Lok Sabha is
(a) One-fourth of the total membership
(b) One-tenth of the total membership
(c) Fifty percent strength of the Lok Sabha
(d) At least hundred members

64. In India which of the following taxes is levied by the State governments?
(a) Excise duty on liquor
(b) Capital gains tax
(c) Customs tax
(d) Corporation tax

65. After hour, a motion moved by a Member of Parliament to draw the attention of Executive for discussing a definite matter of public importance is
(a) Privilege motion
(b) Calling attention Motion
(c) Adjournment motion
(d) No-confidence motion

66. The Chairman of the Public Accounts Committee of the Parliament is appointed by the
(a) President of India
(b) Prime Minister of India
(c) Speaker of Lok Sabha
(d) Chairman of Rajya Sabha

67. Which of the following constitutional Amendment Act, deals with the Elementary Education as a Fundamental Right?
(a) 84th Amendment Act
(b) 85th Amendment Act
(c) 86th Amendment Act
(d) 87th Amendment Act

68. In which way the President can assign any of the functions of the Union Government to the State Government?
(a) In his discretion
(b) In consultation with the Chief Justice of India
(c) In consultation with the Government of the State
(d) In consultation with the State Governor

69. In the 42nd Constitutional Amendment 1976, which word was added to the Preamble?
(a) Democratic (b) Equality
(c) Secular (d) Socialist

70. Chief Ministers of States are members of ________.
(a) NITI Commission(Aayog)
(b) Finance Commission
(c) National Development Council
(d) Election Commission

71. The Comptroller and Auditor General is closely connected with which of the following Committees of Parliament?
(a) The Estimates Committee
(b) The Committee on Public Undertakings
(c) The Public Accounts Committee
(d) All of these

72. The Speaker of Lok Sabha addresses his letter of resignation to the
(a) President of India
(b) Prime Minister
(c) Deputy Speaker of Lok Sabha
(d) The Chief Justice of India

73. The power of the Supreme Court of India to decide disputes between the Centre and the States falls under its
(a) Advisory jurisdiction
(b) Original jurisdiction
(c) Appellate jurisdiction
(d) Jurisprudence

74. If a budget is defeated in the legislature of a state then
(a) The Finance Minister alone has to resign
(b) The Finance Minister concerned has to be suspended
(c) The council of Ministers along with the Chief Minister has to resign
(d) Re-election have to be ordered

75. Lok Sabha Secretariat comes under the direct control of
(a) Ministry of Home Affairs
(b) Ministry of Parliamentary Affairs
(c) Speaker of Lok Sabha
(d) President

76. The word "Secular" was added to the Preamble of the Constitution of India by which Constitutional Amendment?

(a) 41st Constitutional Amendment
(b) 42nd Constitutional Amendment
(c) 43rd Constitutional Amendment
(d) 44th Constitutional Amendment

77. What is the minimum age for membership to Rajya Sabha ?
(a) 20 years (b) 25 years
(c) 30 years (d) 35 years

78. The minimum age limit for the membership of the Vidhan Parishad is _____.
(a) 21 years (b) 25 years
(c) 30 years (d) 35 years

79. The Preventive Detention Act curtailed
(a) Right to Freedom
(b) Right to Equality
(c) Right to Property
(d) Education Right

80. Ideas of welfare state are contained in
(a) Fundamental Rights
(b) Directive Principles of State Policy
(c) Preamble of the Constitution
(d) Part VII

81. Who has the right to decide whether a Bill is a money bill or not?
(a) Speaker of Lok Sabha
(b) Prime Minister
(c) President
(d) Finance Minister

82. The discretionary powers of a Governor is limited in
(a) Appointment of Chief Minister
(b) Dismissal of the Ministry
(c) Dissolution of the Legislative Assembly
(d) Assent to Bills

83. Who is the first law officer of the country?
(a) Chief Justice of India
(b) Attorney General
(c) Law Minister
(d) Solicitor General

84. The Residuary powers of legislation under Indian Constitution rests with
(a) President (b) Prime Minister
(c) Parliament (d) States

85. Appointments for all India Services are made by
(a) UPSC
(b) President
(c) Prime Minister
(d) Parliament

86. Right to Constitutional Remedies comes under _____.
(a) Legal rights
(b) Fundamental rights
(c) Human rights
(d) Natural rights

87. The Comptroller and Auditor-General of India submits his report relating to the accounts of the Union to the ______.
(a) Finance Minister
(b) Prime Minister
(c) President
(d) Chief Justice of the Supreme Court

88. Whose recommendation is mandatory to impeach the President of India from his office before the completion of his/her term?
(a) The Prime Minister
(b) The Speaker of the Lok Sabha
(c) The Chief Justice of India
(d) The two houses of the parliament

89. How many types of writ are there in the Indian Constitution?
(a) 5 (b) 4
(c) 3 (d) 2

90. How many Fundamental Duties are mentioned in Indian constitution?
(a) Five (b) Seven
(c) Nine (d) Eleven

91. Part IV of Constitution of India deals with which of the following?
(a) The Union
(b) The States
(c) Fundamental Rights
(d) Directive Principles of State Policy

92. In Indian Constitution, the method of election of President has been taken from which country?
(a) Britain (b) USA
(c) Ireland (d) Australia

93. What is the literal meaning of the term "Quo-Warranto"?
(a) We command
(b) To forbid
(c) By what authority (or) warrant
(d) None of these

94. Who administers the oath of the President of India?
(a) Governor General of India
(b) Chief Justice of India
(c) Prime Minister of India
(d) Vice President of India

95. Who among the following gave monistic theory of sovereignty?
(a) Austin (b) Darwin
(c) Aristotle (d) Marx

96. Which of the following are constituents of Indian Parliament?
(i) The President
(ii) The Council of States (Rajya Sabha)
(iii) The House of the People (Lok Sabha)
(a) (ii) and (iii)
(b) (i) and (ii)
(c) (i) and (iii)
(d) (i), (ii) and (iii)

97. Who among the following is the executive head of state in India?
(a) Prime Minister
(b) President
(c) Cabinet Secretary
(d) Finance Secretary

98. Which of the following has the supreme command of the Indian Defence Forces?
(a) Prime Minister of India
(b) Defence Minister of India
(c) Council of Ministers of India
(d) President of India

99. Anti-defection law is given in which schedule of Indian constitution?
(a) Second Schedule
(b) Tenth Schedule
(c) Third Schedule
(d) Fourth Schedule

100. Who appoints Governor of a state in India?
(a) Prime Minister of India
(b) Council of Minister
(c) Judge of Supreme Court
(d) President of India

101. What is the literal meaning of 'Certiorari'?
(a) We command
(b) To have the body of
(c) To forbid
(d) To be certified (or) to be informed

102. Who among the following is not a member of any of the two houses of our country?
(a) Prime Minister
(b) Finance Minister
(c) President
(d) Railway Minister

103. Which article of Indian constitution has the provision for National Emergency?
(a) Article 350 (b) Article 352
(c) Article 312 (d) Article 280

104. Fundamental duties are mentioned in which of the following part of Indian Constitution?
(a) Part II (b) Part III
(c) Part V (d) Part IV A

105. What is the minimum age for becoming a Governor of state in India?
(a) 30 years (b) 25 years
(c) 35 years (d) 45 years

106. Which of the following is a feature of federal Government?
(a) Supremacy of Parliament
(b) Supremacy of Judiciary
(c) Division of powers between federal and state Government
(d) Single citizenship

107. Under which article, President of India can proclaim financial emergency?
(a) Article 32 (b) Article 349
(c) Article 360 (d) Article 355

108. Under which article, President of India can proclaim Constitutional Emergency?
(a) Article 32 (b) Article 349
(c) Article 356 (d) Article 360

109. How many members of upper house (Rajya Sabha) can be nominated by President of India?
(a) 10 (b) 12
(c) 14 (d) 16

110. Which of the following is justiciable in nature?
(a) Fundamental Duties
(b) Directive principles of state policy
(c) Fundamental Rights
(d) None of these

111. Which of the following Amendments is also known as the 'Mini Constitution' of India?
(a) 7th Amendment
(b) 42nd Amendment
(c) 44th Amendment
(d) 74th Amendment

112. Which of the following right has been removed from fundamental rights and converted to a simple legal right?
(a) Right to life and personal liberty
(b) Right to property
(c) Right to education
(d) Right to freedom of religion

113. Which of the following does not come under Fundamental Duty?
(a) To safeguard public property
(b) To protect and improve the natural environment
(c) To promote harmony
(d) To protect freedom of speech and expression

114. Comptroller and Auditor General of India is appointed for how many years?
(a) 2 (b) 4
(c) 6 (d) 5

115. Who is the custodian of Contingency Fund of India?
(a) The Prime Minister
(b) Judge of Supreme Court
(c) The President
(d) The Finance Minister

116. Which of the following Country doesn't have a written Constitution?
(a) United Kingdom
(b) Australia
(c) United States of America
(d) Bangladesh

117. In the Indian Parliamentary System, 'Vote on Account' is valid for how many months (except the year of elections)?
(a) 2 months (b) 3 months
(c) 6 months (d) 9 months

118. India has taken the concept of 'Judicial Review' from which country's constitution?
(a) United States
(b) United Kingdom
(c) Canada
(d) Ireland

119. How many times a person can be elected as the President of India?
(a) One time (b) Two times
(c) Three times (d) There is no limit

120. Which article was referred to as the 'the heart and soul' of the constitution by Dr. B.R. Ambedkar?
(a) Article 4 (b) Article 32
(c) Article 28 (d) Article 30

121. Which of the following provision needs a special majority in Parliament?
(a) Change in Fundamental Rights
(b) Creation of New States
(c) Abolition of Legislative Councils in State
(d) Rules and Procedures in Parliament

122. Which of the following is not a fundamental duty?
(a) To abide by constitution and respect the National Flag
(b) To promote harmony and brotherhood
(c) To uphold and protect the sovereignty
(d) Abolition of titles except military and academic

123. Which article can be used by The President of India to declare financial emergency?
(a) Article 32 (b) Article 349
(c) Article 360 (d) Article 365

124. ______ means that the Supreme Court will reconsider the case and the legal issues involved in it.
(a) Original Jurisdiction
(b) Writ Jurisdiction
(c) Appellate Jurisdiction
(d) Advisory Jurisdiction

125. Which amendment of the Constitution of India increased the age of retirement of High Court judges from 60 to 62 years?
(a) 10th (b) 12th
(c) 15th (d) 245th

126. In which of the following cases did the Supreme Court rule that Constitutional Amendments were also laws under Article 13 of the Constitution of India, which could be declared void for being inconsistent with Fundamental Rights?
(a) Keshavanand Bharati Case
(b) Golaknath Case
(c) Minerva Mills Case
(d) Maneka Gandhi Case

127. Which of the following statement(s) is/are not correct for the Ninth Schedule of the Constitution of India?
1. It was inserted by the first amendment in 1951.
2. It includes those laws which are beyond the purview of judicial review.
3. It was inserted by the 42nd Amendment.
4. The laws in the Ninth Schedule are primarily those which pertain to the matters of national security.

Select the correct answer using the code given below :
(a) 1 and 2 (b) 2 and 3
(c) 3 and 4 (d) 3 only

Answers

1. (b)	**2.** (b)	**3.** (b)	**4.** (d)	**5.** (a)	**6.** (c)	**7.** (a)	**8.** (d)	**9.** (b)	**10.** (c)
11. (a)	**12.** (b)	**13.** (c)	**14.** (d)	**15.** (b)	**16.** (c)	**17.** (d)	**18.** (b)	**19.** (b)	**20.** (a)
21. (d)	**22.** (d)	**23.** (a)	**24.** (b)	**25.** (c)	**26.** (a)	**27.** (c)	**28.** (b)	**29.** (a)	**30.** (a)
31. (d)	**32.** (c)	**33.** (d)	**34.** (a)	**35.** (d)	**36.** (a)	**37.** (d)	**38.** (a)	**39.** (b)	**40.** (a)
41. (b)	**42.** (a)	**43.** (c)	**44.** (a)	**45.** (d)	**46.** (a)	**47.** (b)	**48.** (c)	**49.** (b)	**50.** (b)
51. (c)	**52.** (b)	**53.** (b)	**54.** (c)	**55.** (b)	**56.** (a)	**57.** (c)	**58.** (b)	**59.** (a)	**60.** (c)
61. (d)	**62.** (b)	**63.** (b)	**64.** (a)	**65.** (c)	**66.** (c)	**67.** (c)	**68.** (d)	**69.** (c)	**70.** (c)
71. (c)	**72.** (c)	**73.** (b)	**74.** (c)	**75.** (c)	**76.** (b)	**77.** (c)	**78.** (c)	**79.** (a)	**80.** (b)
81. (a)	**82.** (d)	**83.** (b)	**84.** (c)	**85.** (b)	**86.** (b)	**87.** (c)	**88.** (d)	**89.** (a)	**90.** (d)
91. (d)	**92.** (c)	**93.** (c)	**94.** (b)	**95.** (a)	**96.** (d)	**97.** (b)	**98.** (d)	**99.** (b)	**100.** (d)
101. (d)	**102.** (c)	**103.** (b)	**104.** (d)	**105.** (c)	**106.** (c)	**107.** (c)	**108.** (c)	**109.** (b)	**110.** (c)
111. (b)	**112.** (b)	**113.** (d)	**114.** (c)	**115.** (c)	**116.** (a)	**117.** (a)	**118.** (a)	**119.** (d)	**120.** (b)
121. (a)	**122.** (d)	**123.** (c)	**124.** (c)	**125.** (c)	**126.** (b)	**127.** (c)			

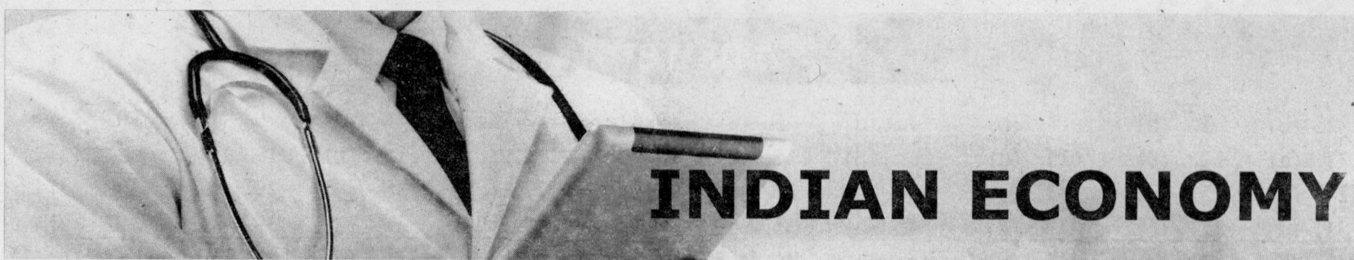

Characteristics of Indian Economy

Main characteristics of Indian economy are:

i. **Agrarian Economy:** In an Agrarian economy, agriculture dominance prevails in both the Gross National Product (GNP) and employment.

ii. **Mixed Economy:** It is an economy, where both public and private sector co-exist.

iii. **Developing Economy:** Following features show that Indian economy is a developing economy:

(a) Low per capita income.

(b) Occupational pattern is primary producing.

(c) Heavy population pressure.

(d) Prevalence of chronic unemployment and under-employment.

(e) Steadily improving rate of capital formation.

(f) Low capital per head.

(g) Unequal distribution of wealth/assets.

Broad Sectors of Indian Economy

- **Primary Sector:** Agriculture forestry, fishing.
- **Secondary Sector:** Mining, manufacturing, electricity gas and water supply, construction.
- **Tertiary Sector:** (also called service sector) Business, transport, telecommunication, banking, insurance, real estate, community and personnel services.

Agriculture and Land Development

Agriculture is the mainstay of the Indian Economy.

Major Crops of India

Types of Crops	Meaning	Major Crops
Foodgrains	Crops that are used for human consumption	Rice, Wheat, Maize, Millets, Pulses and oil seeds
Commercial Crops	Crops which are grown for sale either in raw form or in semi processed form	Cotton, Jute, Sugarcane, Tobacco and oil seeds
Plantation Crops	Crops which are grown on plantations covering large estates	Tea, Coffee, Coconut and Rubber
Horticulture	Sections of agriculture in which fruits and vegetables are grown	Fruits and vegetables

Economic Planning

The Planning Commission was constituted in India in 1950 as a non-constitutional and advisory corporation.

Niti Aayog

- NITI Aayog or National Institution for Transforming India Aayog is the replacement of Planning Commission of India.
- National Institution for Transforming India (NITI) Aayog has been created in accordance to the announcement made by the Prime Minister, Narendra Modi on 15 August, 2014.
- PM is the chairperson of this Niti Aayog.

Major Functions

- An administration paradigm in which the Government is an 'enabler' rather than a 'provider of the first and last resort'.
- Progress from 'food security' to focus on a mix of agricultural production, as well as actual returns that farmers get from their produce.
- To ensure, on areas that are specifically referred to it, that the interests of national security are incorporated in economic strategy and policy.

National Development Council

- National Development Council was constituted on 6 August 1952.
- The Prime Minister is the ex-officio Chairman and the Secretary of Planning Commission is the ex-officio Secretary of this council.
- Chief Ministers of all the states and the members of Planning Commission are the members of National Development Council (NDC). It is an extra-constitutional body.

The Indian Capital Market

- The capital market in India includes: (i) Government Securities (Gilt-edged market); (ii) Industrial Securities Market; (iii) Development financial institutions like IFCI, IDBI, ICICI, SFCs, IIBI, UTI, etc.; and (iv) financial intermediaries like merchant banks.
- Merchant bank, mutual fund, leasing companies, risk capital companies, etc. collect and invest public money into the capital market.
- Unit Trust of India (UTI) is the biggest Mutual Fund Institution of India.

Stock Exchange

- The stock exchanges is the market for buying and selling of stocks, shares, securities, bonds and debentures, etc.
- Under the Securities Contract (Regulation) Act of 1956, the Government of India has so far recognised

23 stock exchanges. Bombay is the premier exchange in the country.

Banking in India

- The Finance Ministry issues currency notes and coins of rupee one, all other currency notes are issued by the Reserve Bank of India.
- The public sector banks account for more than 92% of the entire banking business in India occupying a dominant position in the commercial banking. The State Bank of India and its associate banks along with another 19 banks are the public sector banks.

Establishment of Various Financial Institutions

1.	Reserve Bank of India	1934
2.	Industrial Finance Corporation of India	1948
3.	ICICI	1955
4.	SBI	1955. Nationalised
5.	Life Insurance Corporation (LIC)	1956
6.	Industrial Development Bank of India (IDBI)	1964
7.	Unit Trust of India (UTI)	1964
8.	HUDCO	1970
9.	General Insurance Corporation (GIC)	1972
10.	NABARD	1982
11.	SEBI (Replaced Controller of Capital Issue)	1988. Functional in 1992
12.	Small Industries Development Bank of India (SIDBI)	1990. Subsidiary of IDBI
13.	IRDA	1999

Scheduled and Non-scheduled Banks

- The scheduled banks are those which are entered in the second schedule of the RBI Act, 1934.
- The commercial banks (India and foreign), regional rural banks and state co-operative banks are scheduled banks. Non-scheduled banks are those which are not included in the second schedule of the RBI Act, 1934.

Reserve Bank of India (RBI)

- RBI was set up on the basis of Hilton Young Commission recommendation in April 1935, with the enactment of RBI Act, 1934. Its first Governor was C.D. Deshmukh.
- The headquarters of RBI is in **Mumbai**.

The quantitative credit control consists of:

- **Bank Rate:** It is also called the rediscount rate. It is the rate, at which the RBI gives finance to commercial banks.
- **Cash Reserve Ratio** (CRR): The RBI (Amendment) Bill, 2006, empowers RBI to prescribe CRR–Cash that banks deposit with the RBI without any floor rate or ceiling rate.
- **Statutory Liquidity Ratio** (SLR): It is the ratio of liquid asset, which all commercial Banks have to keep in the form of cash, gold and **unencumbered** approved securities equal to not more than 40% of their total demand and time deposit liabilities (range is 25-40%).
- **Repo Rate:** It is the rate, at which RBI lends short-term money to the bank against securities.
- **Reverse Repo Rate:** It is the rate, at which banks park short-term excess liquidity with the RBI.
- **Open Market Operations** (OMOs): Under OMOs, the RBI sells G-securities in the market.

Regional Rural Banks

The Regional Rural Banks (RRBs), the newest form of banks, have come into existence since middle of 1970s (sponsored by individual nationalised commercial banks) with the objective of developing rural economy by providing, crediting and depositing facilities for agriculture and other productive activities of all kinds in rural areas.

Co-operative Banks

Co-operative banks are so-called because they are organised under the provisions of the Co-operative Credit Societies law of the states. The major beneficiary of the Co-operative Banking is the agricultural sector in particular and the rural sector in general. The first such bank was established in 1904.

Development Banks

- **Industrial Development Bank of India** (IDBI), established in 1964.
- **Industrial Finance Corporation of India** (IFCI), established in 1948.
- **Industrial Credit and Investment Corporation of India Limited** (ICICI), established in 1991.
- **Small Industries Development Bank of India (SIDBI),** established in 1988.
- **Export-Import Bank of India** (Exim Bank), established in 1982.
- National Housing Bank (NHB) started operations in 1988.
- **NABARD** (National Bank for Agriculture and Rural Development) was established in 1982.

Insurance

- Insurance industry includes two sectors–Life Insurance and General Insurance. Life Insurance in India was introduced by Britishers. A British firm in 1818 established the Oriental Life Insurance Company at Calcutta now Kolkata.
- Life Insurance Corporation (LIC) of India was established in September 1956. General Insurance Corporation (GIC) was established in November 1972.

Insurance Regulatory and Development Authority (IRDA)

- IRDA was set up on April 19, 2000 under the IRDA Act, 1999.
- IRDA comprises of a chairman, three whole-time members and four part-time members.

Tax System

- A compulsory contribution given by a citizen or organisation to the government is called Tax.
- There are two types of taxes: 1. Direct Taxes and 2. Indirect Taxes.
- **Direct Taxes:** The taxes levied by the Central Government on income and wealth are important direct taxes. The important taxes levied on incomes are–corporation tax and income tax. Taxes levied on wealth are wealth tax, gift tax, etc.
- **Indirect Taxes:** The main forms of indirect taxes are customs and excise duties and sales tax. The Central Government is empowered to levy customs and excise duties (except on alcoholic liquors and narcotics) where sales tax is the exclusive jurisdiction of the State Governments.
- **Progressive Tax:** A tax that takes away a higher proportion of one's income as the income rises is known as progressive tax. Indian Income Tax is a progressive and direct tax.
- **GST:** GST would be applicable on "supply" of goods or services as against the present concept of tax on the manufacture of goods or on sale of goods or on provision of services. GST would be based on the principle of destination based consumption taxation as against the present principle of origin-based taxation. It would be a dual GST with the Centre and the States simultaneously levying it on a common base. The GST to be levied by the Centre would be called Central GST (central tax-CGST) and that to be levied by the States [including Union territories with legislature] would be called State GST (state tax-SGST). Union territories without legislature would levy Union territory GST (union territory tax-UTGST).

Industry

Industry sector comprises mining, manufacturing, electricity and gas and construction.

Public Sector

In terms of ownership, public sector enterprise (PSE) comprises all undertakings that are owned by the government, or the public, whereas private sector comprises enterprises that are owned by private persons.

Maharatna

In 2009, the government established the **Maharatna** status, which raised the PSEs investment ceiling from ₹ 1,000 crores to ₹ 5,000 crores.

List of Maharatnas

- Oil and Natural Gas Corporation (ONGC)
- Bharat Heavy Electricals Limited (BHEL)
- Gas Authority of India Limited (GAIL)
- Steel Authority India Limited (SAIL)
- Indian Oil Corporation (IOC)
- National Thermal Power Corporation (NTPC)
- Coal India Limited (CIL)
- Bharat Petroleum Corporation Limited.

List of Navratnas

- Bharat Electronics Limited
- Hindustan Aeronautics Limited
- Hindustan Petroleum Corporation Limited
- Mahanagar Telephone Nigam Limited
- National Aluminium Company Limited
- National Mineral Development Corporation
- Neyveli Lignite Corporation Limited
- Oil India Limited
- Power Finance Corporation Limited
- Power Grid Corporation of India Limited
- Rashtriya Ispat Nigam Limited
- Rural Electrification Corporation Limited
- Shipping Carnation of India Limited
- Container Corporation of India Ltd.
- Engineers India Ltd.
- National Building Construction Corporation Ltd.

Navratna

To qualify as a Navratna Company:

- The company must obtain a score of 60 (of the total 100).
- The score is based on six parameters, which included net profit to net worth, total manpower cost to total cost of production, Profit before Depreciation, Interest and Taxes (PBDIT) to capital employed, PBDIT to turnover, earning per share and inter-sectoral performance.
- The company must first be a Miniratna-I and must have four independent directors on its board.
- The Navratna status empowers a company to invest upto ₹ 1,000 crores on 15% of their net worth overseas without government approval.
- At present, there are **16 Navratnas**.

Small Scale Industries

Their importance can be explained as:

i. Employment Generation.
ii. Equitable Distribution.
iii. Mobilisation of Small Savings.
iv. Exports contribution.
v. Environment-friendly.

Large Scale Industries

Iron and Steel Industry

- First steel industry at Kulti, West Bengal–Bengal Iron Works Company was established in 1870.
- First large scale steel plant–TISCO at Jamshedpur (1907) was followed at by IISCO at Burnpur (1919).
- India is the fourth largest producer of crude steel in the world.
- India is the largest producer of sponge iron since 2002.
- Steel Authority of India Limited (SAIL) was established in 1974.

Cotton and Synthetic Textile Industry

It is the largest industry in India. The first Indian modernised cotton cloth mill was established in 1818 at fort Gloster near Kolkata but this was unsuccessful.

Jute Industry

Jute industry was started in 1855 at Resra and India is the largest producer and second largest exporter of jute in the world.

Gems and Jewellery

According to the data released by the World Gold Council (WGC), India is the largest consumer of gold.

Paper Industry

The first paper mill in India was set up at Sreerampur, West Bengal, in the year of 1862.

Silk Industry

- India is the second largest (after China) silk manufacturer.
- The majority of silk is produced mainly in Bhoodan Pochampally (also known as silk city), Kanchipuram, Dharamvaram and Mysore.

Sugar Industry

- India is the largest producer of sugar in the world with a 22% share.

- It is the second largest agro-based industry in the country.
- Dual price mechanism with partial control is applied to sugar industry.

Cement Industry

India is the second largest producer of cement in the world.

Petrochemical Industry

The real thrust to this industry came with the establishment of Indian Petrochemical Corporation Limited at Baroda.

Fertilizer Industry

- The first fertiliser industry was set up in 1906, in **Ranipet** near Chennai.
- India is the third largest producer of fertilizer after China and USA and second largest consumer after China.
- Urea is the only fertilizer under statutory price control.

Automotive Industry

- India is the **second** largest manufacturer of motorcycle and fifth largest manufacturer of commercial vehicles in the world.
- India is the largest manufacturer of tractors in the world.
- Automobile Industry was delicensed in July 1991 with the announcement of the New Industrial Policy.

Steel

- Iron and Steel Industry took birth in India in the year 1870 when Bengal Iron Works Company established its plant at Kulti, West Bengal.
- Large scale iron and steel production was started in 1907 by TISCO established at Jamshedpur (Jharkhand).
- As per the data from International Iron and Steel Institute (IISI) India is the **7th largest producer of steel** in the world.
- At present India is the 9th largest **Crude Steel** producing country in the world.
- Today, India is the largest producer of sponge iron in the world.

Balance of Payments

- BoP comprises current account, capital account and omissions and changes in foreign exchange reserves.
- Under current account transactions are classified into merchandise (exports and imports) and invisibles.
- **Balance of Payment Crisis:** It means that exports exceed imports in value.
- The main component of capital account includes foreign investment, loans and banking capital.

Special Economic Zone (SEZ)

- Asia's first Export Processing Zone (EPZ) was set up in Kandla, India in 1965.
- The first SEZ policy was announced in April 2000.
- SEZ Act, 2005, was enacted with from 10 February 2005.

Exercise

1. The term 'mixed economy' denotes:

(a) existence of both rural and urban sectors
(b) existence of both private and public sectors
(c) existence of both heavy and small industries
(d) existence of both developed and underdeveloped sectors

2. In an economy, the sectors are classified into public and private on the basis of:

(a) employment condition
(b) nature of economic activities
(c) ownership of enterprises
(d) use of raw materials

3. The 'Dual Economy' is a mixture of:

(a) traditional agriculture sector and modern industrial sector
(b) industrial ownership of the manufacturing sector
(c) state ownership of the means of production in corporation of foreign organisation
(d) industrial sector and trading of goods obtained through imports
(e) none of these

4. Which sector of Indian Economy has shown remarkable expansion during the last decade?

(a) Primary Sector
(b) Secondary Sector
(c) Tertiary Sector
(d) Mining Sector

5. When development in economy takes place, the share of tertiary sector in National Income:

(a) first falls and then rises
(b) first rises and then falls
(c) keeps on increasing
(d) remains constant

6. It will be true to classify India as:

(a) A food-deficit economy
(b) A labour-surplus economy
(c) A trade-surplus economy
(d) A capital-surplus economy

7. Mixed economy means:

(a) When agriculture and industry are given equal importance
(b) When public sector exists alongwith the private sector in national economy
(c) Where globalization is transferred with heavy dose of Swadeshi in national economy
(d) Where the centre and the State are equal partners in economic planning and development

8. The Indian Economy is characterised by:

1. Pre-dominance of Agriculture
2. Pre-dominance of Industry
3. Low Per Capita Income
4. Massive Unemployment

Select your answer from the code given below:

Codes:

(a) 1 and 2 only
(b) 1, 2 and 3 only
(c) 2, 3 and 4 only
(d) 1, 3 and 4 only

9. In India, planned economy is based on:

(a) Gandhian System
(b) Socialist System
(c) Capitalist System
(d) Mixed Economy System

10. Economic liberalisation in India started with:
(a) substantial changes in industrial licensing policy
(b) the convertibility of Indian rupee
(c) doing away with procedural formalities for foreign direct investment
(d) significant reduction in tax rates

11. A firm sells new shares worth ₹ 1000 direct to individuals. This transaction will cause:
(a) Gross National Product to rise by ₹ 1000
(b) Gross Domestic Product to rise by ₹ 1000
(c) National Income to rise by ₹ 1000
(d) No impact on Gross National Product

12. Which is not included in the private income arising in a country?
(a) Factor income from net domestic product
(b) Net factor income from abroad
(c) Current transfer from Government
(d) Current payments on foreign loans

13. In India, agriculture income is calculated by:
(a) Output method
(b) Input method
(c) Expenditure method
(d) Commodity method

14. Who coined the term 'Hindu rate of growth' for Indian Economy?
(a) A.K. Sen
(b) Kirit S. Parikh
(c) Raj Krishna
(d) Montek Singh Ahluwalla

15. Under which plan did the Government introduce an agriculture strategy which gave rise to Green Revolution ?
(a) Second Five Year Plan
(b) Third Five Year Plan
(c) Fourth Five Year Plan
(d) Sixth Five Year Plan

16. The Second Five Year Plan was based on:
(a) Mahalanobis Model
(b) Vakil and Brahmanada's Wage — Goods Model
(c) Harrod-Domar Growth Model
(d) Solow Growth Model

17. The Planning Commission of India is:
(a) A constitutional body
(b) An independent and autonomous body
(c) A Statutory body
(d) A non-statutory body

18. Mahalanobis Model has been associated with which Five Year Plan?
(a) First Five Year Plan
(b) Second Five Year Plan
(c) Third Five Year Plan
(d) Fourth Five Year Plan

19. Which plan gave emphasis on removal of poverty for the first time?
(a) Fourth (b) Fifth
(c) Sixth (d) Seventh

20. The period of the Eleventh Five Year Plan is:
(a) 2005 to 2010
(b) 2006 to 2011
(c) 2007 to 2012
(d) 2008 to 2013

21. The Planning Commission of India was constituted in the year:
(a) 1942 (b) 1947
(c) 1950 (d) 1955

22. Which one of the following is NOT correct?
(a) First Five Year Plan: 1951 – 56
(b) Second Five Year Plan: 1956 – 61
(c) Third Five Year Plan: 1961 – 66
(d) Fourth Five Year Plan: 1966 – 71

23. In the post-independence period, economic reformers were first introduced in India under:
(a) Janata Party Government (1977)
(b) Indira Gandhi Government (1980)
(c) Rajiv Gandhi Government (1985)
(d) P.V. Narasimha Rao Government (1990)

24. Only one of the following can be the ex-officio Chairman of the Planning Commission. He is the:
(a) Minister for Planning and Development
(b) Home Minister
(c) Prime Minister
(d) Finance Minister

25. GDP at factor cost is:
(a) GDP minus indirect taxes plus subsidies
(b) GNP minus depreciation allowance
(c) NNP plus depreciation allowances
(d) GDP minus subsidies plus indirect taxes

26. Per Capita Income is obtained by dividing National Income by:
(a) Total population of the country
(b) Total working population
(c) Area of the country
(d) Volume of the capital used

27. Which one of the following is a development expenditure?
(a) Irrigation expenditure
(b) Civil administration
(c) Debt services
(d) Grant-in-Aid

28. Gross Domestic Product (GDP) is defined as the value of all:
(a) goods produced in an economy in a year
(b) goods and services in an economy in a year
(c) final goods produced in an economy in a year
(d) final goods and services product in an economy in a year

29. Depreciation is equal to:
(a) Gross National Product – Net National Product
(b) Net National Product – Gross National Product
(c) Gross National Product – Personal Income
(d) Personal Income – Personal Income

30. Which one of the following is NOT a method of measurement of National Income?
(a) Value Added Method
(b) Income Method
(c) Expenditure Method
(d) Investment Method

31. Net National Product (NNP) of a country is:
(a) GDP minus depreciation allowances
(b) GDP plus net income from abroad
(c) GNP minus net income from abroad
(d) GNP minus depreciation allowances

32. National Income is based on the:
(a) total revenue of the State
(b) production of goods and services

(c) net profit earned and expenditure made by the State
(d) the sum of all factions of income

33. Which of the following is definitely a major indication of the State of the economy of a country?
(a) Rate of GDP growth
(b) Rate of inflation
(c) Number of Banks in a country
(d) Stock of foodgrains in a country

34. Which of the following can be called as a part of the Service Sector?
(a) Textile Mills
(b) Banking
(c) Coal Mines
(d) Agriculture

35. Many a times we read a term in financial newspapers 'GDP'. What is the full form of the same?
(a) Gross Domestic Product
(b) Global Domestic Ratio
(c) Global Depository Receipts
(d) None of these

36. Which sector of Indian Economy contributes largest to the Gross National Product?
(a) Primary Sector
(b) Secondary Sector
(c) Tertiary Sector
(d) Public Sector

37. National Income estimates in India are prepared by:
(a) Planning Commission
(b) Reserve Bank of India
(c) Central Statistical Organisation
(d) Indian Statistical Institute

38. Per Capita Income of country is derived from:
(a) National Income
(b) Population
(c) National Income and Population both
(d) None of these

39. The main source of National Income in India is:
(a) Service Sector
(b) Agriculture
(c) Industrial Sector
(d) Trade Sector

40. The base year for computation of National Income in India is:
(a) 1990 - 91
(b) 1993 - 94
(c) 1999 - 2000
(d) 2000 - 01

41. In India, Hindu Rate of Growth is associated with which of the following?
(a) Birth rate\
(b) Population
(c) Per Capita Income
(d) National Income

Answers

1. (b)	**2.** (c)	**3.** (a)	**4.** (c)	**5.** (c)	**6.** (b)	**7.** (b)	**8.** (d)	**9.** (b)	**10.** (a)
11. (d)	**12.** (d)	**13.** (a)	**14.** (c)	**15.** (b)	**16.** (a)	**17.** (d)	**18.** (b)	**19.** (b)	**20.** (c)
21. (c)	**22.** (d)	**23.** (d)	**24.** (c)	**25.** (a)	**26.** (a)	**27.** (a)	**28.** (d)	**29.** (a)	**30.** (d)
31. (d)	**32.** (b)	**33.** (a)	**34.** (b)	**35.** (a)	**36.** (c)	**37.** (c)	**38.** (c)	**39.** (a)	**40.** (b)
41. (d)									

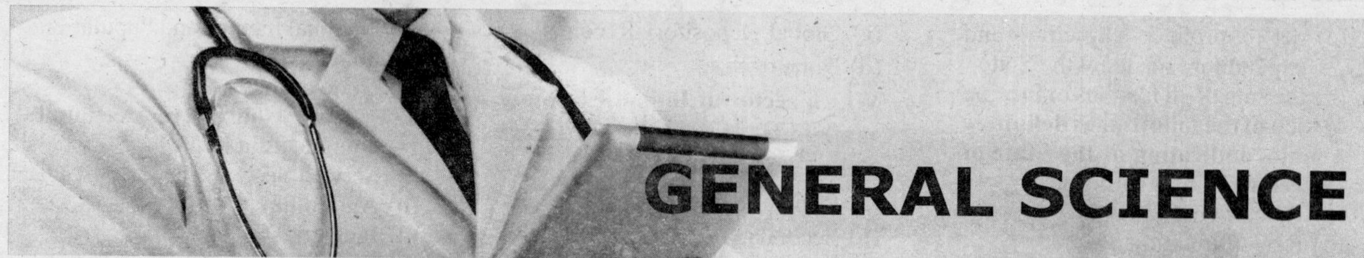

PHYSICS

Unit

The chosen standard used for measuring a physical quantity is called unit.

System of Units

Units depend on choice. Each choice of units leads to a new system (set) of units.

The internationally accepted systems are (i) CGS system; (ii) EPS System; (iii) FPS System; and (iv) SI Units.

SI Base Units

Base quantity	Unit	Symbol
Length	metre	m
Mass	kilogram	kg
Time	second	s
Electric current	ampere	A
Thermodynamic temperature	kelvin	K
Amount of substance	mole	mol
Luminous intensity	candela	cd
Supplementary Physical Quantity	**Supplementary Unit**	**Symbol**
Plane angle	radian	rad.
Solid angle	steradian	Sr

Standard Units

viscocity	pascal second
Power	dioptre
Inductance	henry
Loudness	phon
Magnetic inductance	tesla
Magnetic flux	weber
Electric charge	farad, coulomb

Scalar Quantities

Physical quantities which have magnitude only and no direction are called scalar quantities.

Example: Mass, Speed, Volume, etc.

Vector Quantities

Physical quantities which have magnitude and direction both and which obey triangle law are called vector quantities.

Example: Displacement, Velocity, etc.

Kinematics

Distance

Distance is the length of actual path covered by a moving object in a given time interval.

- Distance is a scalar quantity whereas displacement is a vector quantity both having the same unit (metre).

Displacement

- The difference between the final and the initial position of an object is called displacement. It may be positive, negative or zero.
- It is a vector quantity. Its unit is metre.
- The magnitude of displacement may or may not be equal to the path length traversed by an object.

Speed

- The **average speed** of particle for a given interval of time is defined as the ratio of total distance travelled to the total time taken.

$$\text{Average speed} = \frac{\text{Total distance travelled}}{\text{Total time taken}}$$

- Displacement may be positive, negative or zero whereas distance is always positive.
- Distance travelled by the moving object in unit time interval is called speed. It is scalar quantity and its SI unit is metre/second (m/s). Velocity of a moving object is defined as the displacement of the object in the unit time interval. It is a vector quantity and its SI unit is metre/second.
- Acceleration of an object is defined as the rate of change of velocity of the object. It is a vector quantity and its SI unit is metre/second^2 (m/s^2). If velocity decreases with time then acceleration is negative and is called retardation.

$$\text{Velocity} = \frac{\text{Displacement}}{\text{time}}$$

Uniform Velocity

- An object is said to be moving with uniform velocity if it undergoes equal displacements in equal intervals of time.

Angular Velocity

The angle subtended by the line joining the object from the origin of circle in unit time interval is called angular velocity.

Relative Velocity

- When two bodies are moving in the straight line, the speed (or velocity) of one with respect to another is known as its relative speed (or velocity).

Important Prefixes to Units

tera (T) 10^{12}	giga (G) 10^9	Mega (M)10^6
kilo (K) 10^3	hecto (h) 10^2	deka (da) 10
deci (d) 10^{-1}	centi (C) 10^{-2}	mili (m) 10^{-3}
Micro (μ) 10^{-6}	nano (n) 10^{-9}	Pilo (P) 10^{-12}
Femp (f) 10^{-15}	atto (a) 10^{-18}	

Acceleration

- It is the rate of change of velocity. Its SI unit is m/s^2. It is a vector quantity.
- When the velocity of a body increases with time then its acceleration is negative and is called retardation or deceleration.

Motion

If the position of an object changes with time, it is said to be in motion. A particle at rest does not have the speed and acceleration, while a particle in motion has its speed and also may have some acceleration.

Projectile Motion

- When a particle is so projected that it makes certain angle with horizontal then the motion of the particle is said to be projectile.
- Path of projectile is a parabola.
- To achieve maximum range the body should be projected at an angle of 45°.
- When a body is dropped freely from the top of the tower and another body is projected horizontally from the same point, both will reach the ground at the same time.
- If we throw two balls of different masses in horizontal direction then they will again reach on earth at the same time because both the balls will have zero velocity in vertical direction.

Circular motion

- When an object moves along a circular path, then its motion is called circular motion e.g., motion of a top etc.
- If an object moves a long a circular path with uniform speed, its motion is called uniform circular motion.
- It is accelerated even if speed of the body is constant. The motion of satellite is an acclerated motion.

Newton's first law of motion

- Everybody maintains its initial state of rest or of motion with uniform speed on a straight line unless an external force acts on it.
- First law is also called law of Galileo or law of inertia.

Inertia

Inertia is the property of a body by virtue of which the body opposes change in its initial state of rest or motion with uniform speed on a straight line.

Some Examples of Inertia

- When a car or train starts suddenly, the passengers bend backward.
- When a running horse stops suddenly, the rider bends forward.
- When a coat/blanket is beaten by a stick, the dust particles are removed.
- First law gives the definition of force.

Force

Force is that external cause which when acts to a body changes or tries to change the initial state of the body. Momentum is the property of a moving body and is defined as the product of mass and velocity of the body. It is a vector quantity. Its SI unit is kg m/s.

Newton's Second Law of Motion

- The rate of change in momentum of a body is directly proportional to the applied force on the body and takes place in the direction of force.
- Newton's second law gives the magnitude of force.
- Newton's first law is contained in the second law.

Newton's Third Law of Motion

To every action, there is an equal and opposite reaction.

Centripetal Force

A body performing circular motion is acted upon by a force which is always directed towards the centre of the circle. This force is called centripetal force.

Cyclist bends his body towards the centre on a turn while turning to obtain the required centripetal force.

Centrifugal Force

In applying the Newton's laws of motion, we have to consider some forces which cannot be assigned to any object in the surrounding. These forces are called pseudo force or inertial force. Centrifugal force is also called a Pseudo force. It is always equal and opposite to centripetal force.

Cream separator, centrifugal driver, etc. work on the principle of centrifugal force.

Moment of Force

- The rotational effect of a force on a body about an axis of rotation is described in terms of moment of force.
- The centre of gravity of a body is that point, through which the entire weight of body acts.
- The weight of a body acts through centre of gravity in the downward direction.

Work, Energy and Power

Work

- When a body is displaced by applying a force on it, then work is said to be done.

Positive Work Done

- Positive work means that force is parallel to displacement.

Negative Work Done

- Negative work means that force is opposite to displacement.

Zero Work Done

- If the force is perpendicular to the displacement and if either the force or the displacement is zero, work done is zero.

Energy

- It is defined as capacity of doing work.
- Its unit is joule in SI and erg in CGS system.
- Capacity of doing work by a body is called its energy.
- Energy is a scalar quantity and its SI unit is joule.
- Energy developed in a body due to work done is called mechanical energy.

PE of a body in the gravitational field of earth is *mgh*.
where m = mass, g = acceleration due to gravity, h = height of the body from surface of the earth.

Kinetic Energy

- If a body of mass m is moving with velocity v, then kinetic energy

$$KE = \frac{1}{2}mv^2 = \frac{P^2}{2m}$$

where p is the linear momentum.

- When momentum is doubled, kinetic energy becomes four times.
- If a body is moving in horizontal circle then its kinetic energy is same at all points, but if it is moving in vertical circle, then the kinetic energy is different at different points.

Potential Energy

- It is the energy possessed by a body by virtue of its position.
- Suppose a body is raised to a height h above the surface of the earth, then potential energy of body = *mgh*.
- When a body is falling downwards, then its potential energy goes on changing to kinetic energy.

Transformation of Energy

- In a heat engine, heat energy changes into mechanical energy.
- In the electric bulb, the electric energy is converted into light energy.
- In burning coal, oil, etc., the chemical energy changes to heat energy.
- In solar cell, solar energy changes into electrical energy.
- In playing sitar, mechanical energy changes into sound energy.
- In microphone, sound energy changes into electrical energy.
- In loud speaker, electrical energy changes into sound energy.
- In battery, chemical energy changes into mechanical energy.
- In electric motor, electrical energy changes into mechanical energy.

Power

- Rate of doing work is called power.
- SI unit of power is watt named as a respect to the scientist James Watt or Joule Per second and it is scalar quantity.

  1 W = 1 J/s
  1 kW = 10^3 W
  1 MW = 10^6 W
  1 Watt/s (W–s) = 1 J
- Horse power is a practical unit of power. 1 H.P. = 746 watt.

Power is the rate at which work is done. It is the work/time ratio. Mathematically, it is computed using the following equation:

$$\text{Power} = \frac{\text{Work done}}{\text{Time taken}}$$

$$P = \frac{W}{T}$$

Gravitation

Definition

Every body attracts another body by a force called force of gravitation.

Gravitational Force

- Mathematically, it is represented as: $F = G\frac{Mm}{r^2}$

Where, F is gravitational force, G is gravitational constant, M is the mass of first particle, m is the mass of second particle and r is the distance between them.

- This is called Newton's Universal Law of Gravitation.
- The value of G is 6.67×10^{-11} N m²/kg².

Newton's Law of Gravitation

The force of gravitational attraction between two-point bodies is directly proportional to the product of their masses and inversely proportional to the square of the distance between them.

Gravity

- The acceleration due to gravity is the rate of increase of velocity of a body falling freely towards the earth. It is represented by

$$g = \frac{GM_e}{R_e^2}$$

where $\mathbf{M}_e$ is the mass of the earth and $\mathbf{R}_e$ is the radius of the earth.

- The value of g at the surface of earth is 9.8 m/s².
- The value of g on the Moon is 1/6th of that on the earth.

Variation in the Value of Gravity

- When we go above the surface of the earth, the acceleration due to gravity goes on decreasing.
- When we go below the surface of the earth, the acceleration due to gravity goes on decreasing and becomes zero at the centre of the earth.
- On increasing the rotational motion of earth, the value of g decreases.
- Decreasing the rotational motion of earth, the value of g increases.
- When we go from the equator towards the poles, the value of g goes on increasing.
- If earth stops its rotation about its own axis then at the equator the value of g increases and consequently the weight of body lying there increases.

Variation in g

i. Value of g decreases with height or depth from earth's surface.
ii. g is maximum at poles.
iii. g is minimum at equator.
iv. g decreases due to rotation of earth.
v. g decreases if angular speed of earth increases and increases if angular speed of earth decreases.

- If angular speed of earth becomes 17 times its present value, a body on the equator becomes weightless.

Centre of Gravity

- The centre of gravity of a body is that point at which the whole weight of the body appears to act.
- The gravitational force of earth (gravity) is called acceleration due to gravity (denoted as g) and its value is 9.8 m/s².
- Acceleration due to gravity is independent of shape, size and mass of the body.

Weight

- The weight of a body is the force with which it is attracted towards the centre of Earth.
- It is measured by a spring balance.
- It is not constant and it changes from place to place.

Pressure

- Pressure is defined as force acting normally on unit area on the surface. SI unit of pressure is N/m² also called Pascal (Pa). Pressure is a scalar quantity.

$$\text{Pressure} = \frac{\text{Normal force}}{\text{Area}}$$

- Atmospheric pressure of 1 atm = 1.01 × 10^{-5} N/m² = 760 torr

Atmospheric Pressure

Atmospheric pressure is that pressure which is exerted by a mercury column of 76 cm length at 0°C at 45° latitude at sea-level.

- Atmospheric pressure decreases with altitude (height from earth surface). This is why (i) It is difficult to cook on the mountain. (ii) The fountain pen of a passenger leaks in an aeroplane at a height.
- Atmospheric pressure is measured by barometer.
- Sudden fall in barometric reading is the indication of storm.
- Slow fall in barometric reading is the indication of rain.
- Slow rise in the barometric reading is the indication of clear weathers.

Pressure in liquid

Force exerted on unit area of wall or base of the container by the molecules of liquid is the pressure of liquid.

i. In a static liquid at same horizontal level, pressure is same at all points.
ii. Pressure at a point in a static liquid has same value in all directions.
iii. Pressure at a point in a liquid is proportional to the depth of the point from the free surface.
iv. Pressure at a point in a liquid is proportional to the density of the liquid.

Density

- The density of a substance (ρ) is defined as the ratio of its mass (M) to its volume (V).

i.e. $\text{Density} = \frac{\text{Mass}}{\text{Volume}}$

- Density of water is maximum at 4°C.
- The **relative density** is defined as the ratio of the density of the substance to the density of water at 4°C.
- Ice floats on water surface as its density (0.92 g/cm³) is lesser than the density of water (1g/cm³).
- If ice floating in water in a vessel melts, the level of water in the vessel does not change.
- The density of sea water is more than that of normal water. This explains why it is easier to swim in sea water.

Motion

Simple Harmonic Motion (SHM)

If a particle repeats its motion about a fixed point after a regular time interval in such a way that at any moment the acceleration of the particle is directly proportional to its displacement from the fixed point at the moment and is always directed towards the fixed point at that moment and is always directed towards the fixed point then the motion of the particle is called simple harmonic motion. The fixed point is called mean point or equilibrium point.

Characteristics of SHM

When a particle executing SHM passes through the mean position:

i. No force acts on the particle.
ii. Acceleration of the particle is zero.
iii. Velocity is maximum.
iv. Kinetic energy is maximum.
v. Potential energy is zero.

When a particle executing SHM is at the extreme end, then:

i. Acceleration of the particle is maximum.
ii. Restoring force acting on particle is maximum.
iii. Velocity of particle is zero.
iv. Kinetic energy of a particle is zero.
v. Potential energy is maximum.

Periodic Motion

Any motion which repeats itself after regular interval of time is called periodic or harmonic motion.

Oscillatory Motion

- If a particle repeats its motion after a regular time interval about a fixed point, motion is said to be oscillatory or vibratory.
- Motion of piston in an automobile engine and motion of balance wheel of a watch are the examples of oscillatory motion.

Time Period

Time taken in one complete oscillation is called time period.

Frequency is the number of oscillations completed by oscillating body in unit time interval. Its SI unit is Hertz.

Simple Pendulum

- It is a heavy point mass suspended from a rigid support by means of an elastic inextensible string.
- Time period of simple pendulum $= T = 2\pi\sqrt{\frac{l}{g}}$
- Where l is the length of simple pendulum and g is the acceleration due to gravity.
- If a simple pendulum is suspended in a lift descending down with acceleration, then time period of pendulum will increase. If lift is ascending, then time period of pendulum will decrease.
- If a lift falling freely under gravity, then the time period of the Pendulum will be infinite.

Wave

- A wave is a disturbance which propagates energy from one place to the other without the transport of matter.
- These are of two types:
  i. Mechanical waves
  ii. Electromagnetic waves

Mechanical Waves

- The waves which require material medium (solid, liquid or gas) for their propagation are called mechanical waves or elastic waves.

These are of two types:

i. Longitudinal waves
ii. Transverse waves

Longitudinal Waves: If the particles of the medium vibrate in the direction of propagation of wave, the wave is called longitudinal wave. Waves on springs or sound waves in air are examples of longitudinal waves.

Transverse Waves: If the particles of the medium vibrate perpendicular to the direction of propagation of wave, the wave is called transverse wave.

Waves on strings under tension, waves on the surface of water are examples of transverse waves.

Electromagnetic waves

- The waves which do not require medium for their propagation, i.e. which can propagate even though the vacuum are called non-mechanical waves. Light and heat are the examples of non-mechanical wave. In fact all the electromagnetic waves are non-mechanical.

- All the electromagnetic waves consist of photons.
- The wavelength range of electromagnetic waves is 10^{-4} m to 10^{4} m.

Properties of Electromagnetic Waves

Following waves are not electromagnetic:

i. Cathode rays
ii. Canal rays
iii. Sound waves
iv. Ultrasonic waves

Note: Electroı. agnetic waves of wavelength range 10^{-3} m to 10^{-2} m are called microwaves.

Sound Wave

- It is longitudinal mechanical.
- The longitudinal mechanical waves which lie in the range 20 Hz to 20,000 Hz are called **audible** or **sound waves.**
- The longitudinal mechanical waves having frequencies less than 20 Hz are called **infrasonic**. These are produced by earthquakes, volcanic, eruption, Ocean waves, elephants, and whales.
- The longitudinal mechanical waves having frequencies greater than 2000 Hz are called **ultrasonic waves.**

Applications of Ultrasonic Waves

1. For sending signals.
2. For measuring the depth of sea.
3. For cleaning clothes, aeroplanes and machinery parts of clocks.
4. For removing lamp-shoot from the chimney of factories.
5. In sterilising of a liquid.
6. In ultrasonography.

Speed of Sound

- In a medium, the speed of sound basically depends upon elasticity and density of medium.
- When sound enters from one medium to another medium, its speed and wavelength changes but frequency remains unchanged.
- In a medium the speed of sound is independent of frequency.
- Speed of sound is maximum in solids and minimum in gases.
- The speed of sound is more in humid air than in dry air because the density of humid air is less than the density of dry air.
- The unit of loudness is decibel (dB).

Effect of pressure on speed of sound: The speed of sound is independent of pressure.

Effect of temperature on speed of sound: The speed of sound increases with the increase of temperature of the medium.

Intensity of Sound

Area Code	Kind of area	Intensity during the day (decibel)	Intensity at night (decibel)
A	Industrial area	75	70
B	Commercial area	65	55
C	Residential area	55	45
D	Peaceful area	50	40

Effect of humidity on speed of sound: The speed of sound is more in humid air than in dry because the density of humid air is less than the density of dry air.

Heat

Heat is that form of energy which flows from one body to other body due to difference of temperature between the bodies. The amount of heat contained in a body depends upon the mass of the body.

- It is due to the kinetic energy of the molecules constituting the body.
- Its units are calorie (cal), kilocalorie (kcal) or joule (J).
- 1 cal = 4.18 Joule, 1 kcal = 1000 cal

Temperature

Temperature is that physical cause which decides the direction of flow of heat from one body to other body. Heat energy always flows from body at higher temperature to body at lower temperature.

- The normal temperature of a human body is 37°C or 98.4 °F.
- Triple point is the state at which all the three states of matter co-exist. The triple point of water is 273.16 K.

The device which measures the temperature of a body is called thermometer.

Thermometers

Scale	Minimum Temperature	Maximum Temperature (Boiling Point)
Centigrade or celsius	0°C	100°C
Fahrenheit	32°F	212°F
Reumer	0°R	80°R

Transmission of Heat

Conduction

In this process, heat is transferred from one place to other place by the successive vibrations of the particles of the medium without bodily movement of the particles of the medium. In solids, heat transfer takes place by conduction.

Convection

In this process, heat is transferred by the actual movement of particles from one place to other place. Due to movement of particles, a current of particles sets up, which is called convection current. In liquids and gases, heat transfer takes place by convection.

- Earth's atmosphere is heated by convection.

Radiation

In this method, transfer of heat takes place with the speed of light without affecting the intervening medium.

Fusion

The process by which a substance is changed from solid state to liquid state is called fusion. Fusion takes place at a fixed temperature called melting point (MP).

Freezing

The process by which a substance is changed from liquid state to solid state is called freezing. Freezing takes at a fixed temperature called freezing point (FP). For a substance MP = FP.

- ➤ Melting point of substances which contract in the process of fusion (as ice) decreases with the increase in pressure. Melting point of substances which expand in the process of fusion (as wax) increases with the increase in pressure.
- ➤ With the addition of impurity (as salt in ice), melting point of a substance decreases.

Vapourisation

The process by which a substance is changed from liquid state to vapour state is called vapourisation.

Evaporation

The process of vapourisation which takes place only from the exposed surface of liquid and that at all temperatures is called evaporation.

Evaporation causes cooling. This is why water in an earthen pot gets cooled in summer.

Boiling

The process of vapourisation which takes place at a fixed temperature and from whole part of liquid is called boiling. The temperature at which boiling takes place is called **boiling point**.

Condensation

The process by which a substance is changed from vapour state to liquid state is called condensation.

- ➤ Boiling point of a liquid increases with the increase in pressure.
- ➤ Boiling point of a liquid increases with the addition of impurity.

Light

Light is a form of energy which is propagated as electromagnetic waves. In the spectrum of electromagnetic waves it lies between ultra-violet and infra-red region and has wavelength between 3900 Å to 7800 Å.

- ➤ Electromagnetic waves are transverse, hence light is transverse wave.
- ➤ Wave nature of light explains rectilinear propagation, reflection, refraction, interference, diffraction and polarisation of light.
- ➤ Clearly light behaves as wave and particle both.
- ➤ Speed of light is maximum in vacuum and air (3×10^8 m/s).
- ➤ It is a transverse wave.
- ➤ It takes 8 min 19 s to reach on the earth from the sun.
- ➤ The light reflected from moon takes 1.28 s to reach earth.

Refractive Index

Refractive Index of a medium is defined as the ratio of speed or light in vacuum to the speed of light in the medium.

- ➤ Velocity of light is larger in a medium which has small refractive index.
- ➤ Light takes 8 minute 19 second (499 second) to reach from sun to the earth.
- ➤ The light reflected from moon takes 1.28 second to reach earth.

Luminous Bodies

Those objects which emit light by themselves are called luminous bodies.

Non-luminous Bodies

Those objects which do not emit light by themselves but are visible by the light falling on them emitted by the luminous bodies are called non-luminous bodies.

A material can be classified as:

1. **Transparent:** The bodies which allow most of the incident light to pass through them are called transparent bodies, e.g., glass and water.
2. **Translucent:** The bodies which allow a part of incident light to pass through them are called translucent bodies, e.g., pied paper.
3. **Opaque:** The substances which do not allow the incident light to pass through them are called opaque bodies, e.g., mirror, metal, wood, etc.

Reflection of Light

- ➤ The return of light into the same medium after striking a surface is called reflection.

There are two laws of reflection.

- i. The angle of incidence is always equal to angle of reflection.
- ii. The incident ray, normal and reflected ray, all lie in the same plane.

Reflection From Plane Mirror

- i. The image is virtual and laterally inverted.
- ii. The size of image is equal to that of object.
- iii. The distance of image from the mirror is equal to distance of object from the mirror.
- iv. If an object moves towards (or away from) a plane mirror with speed u, relative to the object, the image moves towards (or away) with a speed of $2v$.
- v. If a plane mirror is rotated by an angle θ, keeping the incident ray fixed, the reflected ray is rotated by an angle 2θ.
- vi. To see his full image in a plane mirror, a person requires a mirror of at least half of his height.

☞ **Note:** Image formed by a convex mirror is always virtual, erect and diminished.

Reflection at spherical surface

- ➤ Spherical mirrors are the mirrors in which reflecting surface side is spherical.

There are two types of spherical mirrors:

- i. convex mirror
- ii. concave mirror

Mirror formula is given by $\frac{1}{v}+\frac{1}{u}=\frac{1}{f}$

u = Object distance

v = Image distance

f = Focal length of the mirror.

Uses of Concave Mirror

- i. As a shaving glass.
- ii. As a reflector for the headlights of a vehicle, search light.
- iii. In ophthalmoscope to examine eye, ear, nose by doctors.
- iv. In solar cookers.

Uses of Convex Mirror

- i. As a rear view mirror in vehicles because it provides the maximum rear field of view and image formed is always erect.
- ii. In sodium reflector lamp.

Image formation by concave mirror

Position of object	Position of image	Size of image	Nature of image
At infinity	At F	Highly diminished	Real and inverted
Between infinity and C	Between F and C	Diminished	"
At C	At C	Same size	"
Between F and C	Between infinity and C	Enlarged	"
At F	At infinity	Highly enlarged	"
Between F and P	Behind the mirror	Enlarged	Virtual and erect

Where (C) is centre of curvature
P is pole of the mirror
F is focus.

Image formation by convex mirror

Position of object	Position of image	Size of image	Nature of image
At infinity	At F	Highly dimished	Erect and virtual
Between infinity and Pole	Between F and P	Diminished	Erect and virtual

Refraction of Light

When a ray of light propagating in a medium enters the other medium, it deviates from its path. This phenomenon of change in the direction of propagation of light at the boundary, when it passes from one medium to other medium, is called refraction of light.

When a ray of light enters from rarer medium to denser medium from water to glass) it deviates towards the normal drawn on the boundry of two media at the incident point. Similarly, in passiing from denser to rarer medium, a ray deviates away from the normal. If light is incident normally on the boundary, i.e. parallel to normal, it enters the second medium undeviated.

Laws of Refraction

i. Incident ray, refracted ray and normal drawn at incident point always lie in the same plane.
ii. **Snell's law:** For a given colour of light, the ratio of sine of angle of incidence to the sine of angle of refraction is a constant.

- The refractive index of a medium decreases with the increase in wavelength of light.
- The refractive index of a medium decreases with an increase in temperature.
- When a ray of light enters from one medium to other medium, its frequency and phase do not change but wavelength and velocity changes.

Some Illustrations of Refraction

i. Bending of a linear object when it is partially dipped in a liquid inclined to the surface of the liquid.
ii. Twinkling of stars.
iii. Oval shape of sun in the morning and evening.
iv. An object in a denser medium, when seen from a rarer medium, appears to be at a smaller distance.

- **Due to refraction,** rivers appear shallow, coin in a beaker filled with water appears raised, pencil in the beaker appears broken.
- At sunset and sunrise, due to refraction, **sun appears above horizon** while it is actually below horizon.
- The duration of day appears to be increased by nearly 4 minute to **atmospheric refraction.**
- Writing on a **paper appears lifted** when a glass slab is placed over the paper.
- The refractive index of a medium is maximum for violet colour of light and minimum for red colour of light.
- Refractive index decreases with rise in the temperature.

Critical angle: In case of propagation of light from denser to rarer medium through a plane boundary, critical angle is the angle of incidence for which angle of refraction is 90°.

Total Internal Reflection of Light

- If the angle of incidence in denser medium is greater than critical angle (*C*), then the ray is reflected back into the first rarer medium, this phenomenon is called **total internal reflection.**
- In a desert, the phenomenon of **mirage** occurs due to total internal reflection.

Illustrations of Total Internal Reflection

i. Sparkling of diamond.
ii. Mirage and looming.
iii. Shining of air bubble in water.
iv. Increase in duration of sun's visibility.
v. Shining of a smoked ball or a metal ball on which lamp stool deposited when dipped in water.
vi. Optical Fibre.

Applications

i. For transmitting optical signals and the two dimensional picture.
ii. For transmitting electrical signals by first converting them to light.
iii. For visualising the internal sites of the body by doctors in endoscopy.

Refraction of Light through Lens

- When a lens is thicker at the middle than at the edges, it is called convex lens or a converging lens. When the lens is thicker at edge than in the middle, it is called as concave lens or diverging lens.

lenses

- Lens is a transparent medium bounded by two curved surfaces. Lenses are of two types:

i. Concave or divergent lens.
ii. Convex or convergent lens

$$\text{Magnification } (m) = \frac{\text{Lenght (height) of image}}{\text{Length (height) of object}} = \frac{v}{u}$$

Image Formation by a Convex Lens

Position of object	Position of image	Size of image	Nature of image
At infinity	At F_2	Highly diminished	Real and inverted
Beyond 2 F_1	Between F_2 and 2 F_2	Diminished	Real and inverted
At 2 F_1	At 2 F_2	Same size	Real and inverted
Between 2 F_1 and F_1	Beyond 2 F_2	Enlarged	Real and inverted
At F_1	At infinity	Highly enlarged	Real and inverted
Between F_1 and lens	Behind the object on the same side of the object	Enlarged	Virtual and erect

Power of a Lens

Power of a lens is its capacity to deviate a ray. It is measured as the reciprocal of the focal length in metres. Unit of power is dioptre (D).

- Power of a convex lens is positive and that of a concave lens is negative.
- If two lenses are placed in contact, then the power of combination is equal to the sum of powers of individual lenses.

Dispersion of Light

When a ray of white light (or a composite light) is passed through a prism, it gets splitted into its constituent colours. This phenomenon is called dispersion of light. The coloured pattern obtained on a screen after dispersion of light is called spectrum.

- The dispersion of light is due to different deviation suffered by different colours of light. The deviation is maximum for violet colour and minimum for red colour of light. The different colours appeared in the spectrum are in the following order: violet, Indigo, Blue, Green, Yellow, Orange and red (VIBGYOR).
- The dispersion of light is due to different velocities of light of different colours in a medium. As a result, the refractive index of a medium is different for different colours of light.
- The velocity of light in a medium is maximum for that colour for which refractive index is minimum.

Rainbow

Rainbow is formed due to dispersion of sun light by the suspended water droplets.

- Primary rainbow is formed due to two refractions and one total internal reflection of light falling on the raindrops.
- Secondary rainbow is formed due to two refractions and two internal reflections of light falling on raindrops.

Human Eye

- Least distance of distinct vision is 25 cm.

Defects of Human Eye and the Remedies

1. **Myopia or short sightedness:** A person suffering from myopia can see the near objects clearly while far objects are not clear.
   Remedy: Diverging lens is used.
2. **Hyperopia or hypermetropia or longsightedness:** A person suffering from hypermetropia can see the distant objects clearly but not the near objects.
   Remedy: A converging lens is used.
3. **Presbyopia:** This defect is generally found in elderly person. Due to stiffening of ciliary muscles, eye looses much of its accommodating power. As a result, the distant as well as the nearby objects cannot be seen.
   Remedy: For its remedy, two separate lenses or a bifocal lens are/is used.
4. **Astigmatism:** This defect arises due to difference in the radius of curvature of cornea in the different planes. As a result rays from an object in one plane are brought to focus by eye in another plane. For its remedy cylindrical lens is used.

Electricity

Charge

Charge is the basic property associated with matter due to which it produces and experiences electric and magnetic effects.

- It is something that a body attains when it loses or gains the electrons.
- Its S.I. unit is coulomb C.
- Electricity is associated with the charge.
- Similar charges repel each other and opposite charges attract each other.
- The proton possesses positive charge (+ e) and electron possesses an equal negative charge (– e).
- Charging of bodies takes place due to transfer of electrons from one body to other body.
- Human body and earth act like a conductor. Silver is the best conductor.
- The surface density of charge at a point on the surface of conductor depends upon the shape of conductor and presence of other conductors or insulators near the given conductor.
- The surface density of charge at any part of the conductor is inversely proportional to the radius of curvature of the surface of that part.

This is why surface density of charge is maximum at the pointed parts of the conductor.

Conductor

Conductors are those materials which allow electricity (charge) to pass through them.

Examples: (a) Metals like silver, iron, copper, (b) Earth (especially the most part) acts like a huge conductor.

Insulator or Dielectric: Insulators are those materials which do not allow electricity to flow through them.

Examples: Wood, paper.

> **Coulomb's Law**
> According to Coulomb's law, the attraction or repulsion between two point charges at rest is directly proportional to the product of the magnitudes of the charges and inversely proportional to the square of the distance between them.

Electric Field

- The region around an electric charge in which the electric effect can be experienced is called the electric field.
- Electric field intensity inside a charged hollow conductor is zero.

Electric Field Intensity

Electric field intensity at a point in an electric field is the force experienced by a unit positive charge placed at that point.

Electric Field of hollow conductor: Electric field intensity inside a charged hollow conductor is zero. Charge given to such a conductor (or conductor of any shape) remains on its surface only.

This explains why a hollow conductor acts as an electrostatic shield. For this reason it is safer to sit in a car or bus during lightning.

Electric Potential: Electric potential at a point in an electric field is the work done in bringing a unit positive charge from infinity to that point. SI unit of electric potential is volt.

Potential Difference: Work done in bringing a unit positive charge from one point to other point is the potential difference between the two points. Its SI unit is volt and it is a scalar quantity.

Electric Capacity

Electric capacity of a conductor is defined as the charge required to increase the potential of the conductor by unity. Its SI unit is farad (F).

Electric Current

Electric current is defined as the rate of flow of charge or charge flowing per unit time interval. Its direction is the direction of flow of positive charge. Its SI unit is ampere (A).

Resistance: The opposition offered by a conductor to the flow of current through it is called resistance. Its SI unit is ohm.

Ohm's Law

If physical conditions like temperature, intensity of light, etc. remains unchanged then electric current flowing through a conductor is directly proportional to the potential difference across its ends.

Ohmic Resistance: The resistances of such conductors which obey Ohm's law are called ohmic resistances. For example, resistance of melanin wire.

Non-ohmic Resistance: The resistances of such materials which do not obey ohm's law are called non-ohmic resistances.

Example: Resistance of diode valve, resistance of triode valve.

Conductance

Reciprocal of resistance of a conductor is called its conductance.

Its SI unit is ohm^{-1} (also called mho or siemen.)

- The resistance of a conductor is directly proportional to its length and inversely proportional to its cross sectional area.

Specific conductance or conductivity: The reciprocal of resistivity of a conductor is called its conductivity (s). Its SI unit is mho m^{-1} or siemen metre (sm^{-1}).

- In series combination, the equivalent resistance is equal to the sum of the resistances of individual conductors. ($R = R_1 + R_2 + ...R_n$)
- In parallel combination, the reciprocal of equivalent resistance is equal to the sum of the reciprocal of individual resistances.
- **Specific resistance** or **Resistivity** depends only on the material of conductor and its temperature. Resistivity increases with temperature.
- If a wire is stretched or doubled on itself, its resistance will change, but its specific resistance will remain unaffected.

Electric Power

The rate at which electrical energy is consumed in a circuit is called electric power. Its SI unit is watt.

1 kilowatt hour = 3.6×10^6 joule

Ammeter

Ammeter is a device which is used to measure electric current in a circuit. It is connected in series in the circuit.

- The resistance of an ideal ammeter is zero.

Voltmeter

Voltmeter is a device used to measure the potential difference between two points in a circuit. It is connected in parallel to the circuit.

- The resistance of an ideal voltmeter is infinite.

Electric Fuse

Electric fuse is a protective device used in series with an electric appliance to save it from being damaged due to high current. In general, it is a small conducting wire of alloy of copper, tin and lead, having low melting point.

- Pure fuse is made up of tin.

Galvanometer

Galvanometer is a device used to detect and measure electric current in a circuit.

Magnetism

- Magnet is a piece of iron or other material that can attract iron containing objects and that points north and south when suspended.

Directive Property

When a magnet is freely suspended, it aligns itself in the geographical north-south direction.

- Natural magnet is oxide of iron.
- The magnets made by artificial methods are called artificial magnets or manmade magnets. They may be of different types like bar magnet, horse shoe magnet, Robinson's ball ended magnet, magnetic needle, electromagnet, etc.
- The two points near the two ends of a magnet where the attracting capacity is maximum are called magnetic poles.
- The imaginary line joining the two poles of a magnet is called magnetic axis of the magnet.
- Similar poles repel each other and dissimilar poles attract each other.

- When magnetic substance is placed near a magnet, it gets magnetised due to induction.

Magnetic Field

Region in space around a magnet where the magnet has its magnetic effect is called magnetic field of the magnet.

Intensity of Magnetic Field or Magnetic Flux Density

Magnetic flux density of a point in a magnetic field is the force experienced by a north pole of unit strength placed at that point.

Its SI unit is Newton/ampere-metre Weber/metre or tesla (T).

Magnetic Lines of Force

The magnetic lines of force are imaginary current which represent a magnetic field graphically.

Magnetic Substance

i. **Diamagnetic substance:** Diamagnetic substances are such substances which, when placed in a magnetic field, acquire feeble magnetism opposite to the direction of the magnetic field.

Examples: Bismuth, Zinc, Copper.

ii. **Paramagnetic Substance:** Paramagnetic substances are such substances which when placed in a magnetic field acquire a feedback magnetised in the direction of field.

Examples: Iron, Cobalt.

Curie Temperature

As temperature increases, the magnetic property of ferromagnetic substance decreases and above a certain temperature the substance changes into paramagnetic substance. This temperature is called Curie temperature.

- Permanent magnets are made of steel, cobalt steel, alcomax or alnico.
- Electromagnets, cores of transformers, telephoediaphragms and motors are made of soft iron, mu-metal and stalloy.

Terrestrial Magnetism

Our earth behaves as a powerful magnet whose south pole is near the geographical North Pole and whose North Pole is near the geographical South Pole.

i. **Declination:** The acute angle between magnetic meridian and geographical meridian at a place is called the angle of declination at that place.

ii. **Dip or Inclination:** Dip is the angle which the resultant earth's magnetic field at a place makes with the horizontal. At poles and equator, dip is 90° and 0° respectively.

List of Scientific Instruments

Instrument	Use
Altimeter	It measures altitudes and is used in aircrafts.
Ammeter	It measures strength of electric current (in amperes).
Anemometer	It measures force and velocity of wind.
AudioPhone	It is used for improving imperfect sense of hearing.
Audiometer	It measures intensity of sound.
Barometer	It measures atmospheric pressure.
Binocular	It is used to view distant objects.
Bolometer	It measures heat radiation.
Barograph	It is used for continuous recording of atmospheric pressure.
Cinematography	It is an instrument used in cinema-making to throw on screen and enlarged image of photograph.
Crescograph	It measures the growth in plants.
Cyclotron	A charged particle accelerator which can accelerate charged particles to high energies.
Calorimeter	It measures quantity of heat.
Carburetor	It is used in an internal combustion engine for charging air with petrol vapour.
Cardiogram	It traces movements of the heart, recorded on a cardiograph.
Chronometer	It determines longitude of a place kept onboard ship.
Dynamometer	It measures electrical power.
Dynamo	It converts mechanical energy into electrical energy.
Endoscope	It examines internal parts of the body.
Eudiometer	Glass tube for measuring volume changes in chemical reactions between gases.
Electrometer	It measures electricity.

Electroscope	It detects presence of an electric charge.
Fathometer	It measures the depth of the ocean.
Galvanometer	It measures the electric current of low magnitude.
Hydrometer	It measures the specific gravity of liquids.
Hygrometer	It measures humidity in air.
Hydrophone	It measures sound under water.
Kymograph	It graphically records physiological movements (blood pressure and heartbeat).
Lactometer	It determines the purity of milk.
Manometer	It measures the pressure of gases.
Mariner's Compass	It is an instrument used by the sailors to determine the direction.
Microphone	It converts the sound waves into electrical vibrations and to magnify the sound.
Microscope	It is used to obtain magnified view of small objects.
Photometer	The instrument compares the luminous intensity of the source of light.
Periscope	It is used to view objects above sea level (used in submarines).
Potentiometer	It is used for comparing electromotive force of cells.
Odometer	An instrument by which the distance covered by wheeled vehicles is measured.
Pyrometer	It measures very high temperature.
Radar	It is used for detecting the direction and range of an approaching plane by means of radio microwaves.
Radiometer	It measures the emission of radiant energy.
Refractometer	It measures refractive index.
Saccharimeter	It measures the amount of sugar in the solution.
Seismograph	It measures the intensity of earthquake shocks.
Speedometer	It is an instrument placed in a vehicle to record its speed.
Sphygmomanometer	It measures blood pressure.
Spherometer	It measures the curvatures of surfaces.
Stereoscope	It is used to view two dimensional pictures.
Sextant	This is used by navigators to find the latitude of a place by measuring the elevation above the horizon of the sun or another star.
Spectrometer	It is an instrument for measuring the energy distribution of a particular type of radiation.
Stethoscope	An instrument which is used by the doctors to hear and analyze heart and lung sounds.
Tachometer	An instrument used in measuring speeds of aeroplanes and motorboats.
Telescope	It views distant objects in space.
Thermometer	This instrument is used for the measurement of temperatures.
Thermostat	It regulates the temperature at a particular point.

Invention and Discovery

Inventions/ Discoveries	Name of the Scientist/Person
Archimedean Screw	Archimedes
Atom	Neils Bohr
Atomic Number	Mosley
Atomic Physics	Enrico Fermi
Atomic Structure	Bohr and Rutherford
Atomic Theory	Dalton

Automatic Gearbox	Hermann Fottinger
Adding Machine	Pascal
Aeroplane	Wright brothers
Air Brake	George Westinghouse
Air Pump	Otto von Guericke
Airship (rigid)	G. Ferdinand von Zeppelin
Aniline Dyes	Hoffman
Antiseptic Surgery	Lord Joseph Lister
Arc Lamp	C. F. Brush
Automobile	Daimler
Automobiles using gasoline	Karl Benz
Avogadro's Hypothesis	Avogadro
Bacteriology	Robert Koch
Bakelite	Leo H Baekeland
Balloon	Jacques and Joseph Montgolfier
Ball-Point Pen	John J. Loud
Barometer	Evangelista Torricelli
Beri-Beri	Eijkman
Bicycle	Kirkpatrick Macmillan
Bicycle Tyre	J.B. Dunlop
Bacteriophage	Max Delbruck
Bifocal Lens	Benjamin Franklin
Binomial Nomenclature	Carl Linnaeus
Biogenetic Principle	Ernst Haeckel
Bismuth	Valentine
Bomb	Edward Teller
Boson	S.N.Bose
Boyle's law	Boyle
Braille	Louis Braille
Breaking up the Nucleus of an atom	Rutherford
Cinema	A.L. and J.L. Lumiere
Centrigrade scale	A. Celsius
Chemical Structure	August Kekule
Chemotherapy	Paul Ehrlich
Chloroform	James Harrison and James Young Simpson
Cholera Bacillus	Robert Koch
Calculating Machine	Pascal
Camera	George Eastman
Carburettor	Gottlieb Daimler
Cell Doctrine	Rudolf Virchow
Celluloid	A. Parker
Cement	Joseph Aspdin
Chromosomal Theory of Heredity	Thomas Hunt Morgan
Chronometer	John Harrison

Cine Camera	Friese-Greene
Cinematography	Thomas Alva Edison
Classical Field Theory	Michael Faraday
Clock (machanical)	Hsing and Ling-Tsan
Clock (pendulum)	C. Hugyens
Coloured Photography	Lippman
Computer	Charles Babbage
Cosmic Rays	R.A.Millikan
Crescograph	J.C.Bose
Crystal Dynamics	C.V.Raman
Cyclotron	Lawrence
Deuterium (Heavy Water)	H.C. Urey
Diesel Engine	Rudolf Diesel
Diesel Oil Engine	Rudolf Diesel
Difference Engine	Charles Babbage
Electrons	J.J. Thomson
Solar System	Copernicus (1540)
Specific Gravity	Archimedes
Dynamite	Alfred B. Nobel
Dynamo	Michael Faraday
Effect of Pressure on Trough Bodies	Meghnad Saha
Eightfold Way	Murray Gell-Mann
Electric Battery	Alessandro Volta
Electrical Waves	Heitz
Electricity	Faraday
Electromagnet	William Sturgeon
Electromagnetic Field	James Clerk Maxwell
Electromagnetic Theory	Maxwell
Electron	Joseph J. Thomson
Electron Theory	Bohr
Electronic Computer	Dr. Alan M. Turing
Elevator	Elisha G. Otis
Energy of the Sun	Hans Bethe
'Equal' sign (=)	Robert Recorde
Ethology	Konrad Lorenz
Eugenics	Francis Galton
Fahrenheit Scale	Fahrenheit
Film and Goods Photographic	Kodak
Electric Flat Iron	H.W. Seeley
Electric Furnace	William Siemens
Electric Generator	Michael Faraday
Electric Guitar	Adolph Rickenbacker
Electric iron	H.W. Seeley
Electric Lamp	Thomas Alva Edison
Electric Measurement	Gauss

Electric Motor (AC)	Nikola Tesla
Electric Razor	Jacob Schick
Film (with sound)	Dr. Lee de Forest
Fundamental Laws of Electric Attraction	Coulomb
Galvanometer	Andre-Marie Ampere
Gas Lighting	William Murdoch
Gasoline Engine	Karl Benz
Genetic Code	Frederick Sanger
Glider	Sir George Caley
Gramophone	Thomas Alva Edison
Gun Powder	Rogei Bacon
Heavens	William Herschel
Heavy Hydrogen	Urey
Helicopter	Broquett
Heliocentric Universe	Nicolaus Copernicus
Helium Gas	Lockyer
Hovercraft	Christopher Cockerell
Hydrogen	Cavendish
Hydrophobia	Louis Pasteur
Intelligence Test	Binet
Internal Combustion Engine	Otto
Jeans	Levi Strauss
Jet Engine	Sir Frank Whittle
Jet Propulsion	Frank Whittle
Kala-azar Fever	U.N. Brahmachari
Kaleidoscope	David Brewster
Laboratory Gas Burner	Robert Wilhelm von Bunsen
I.Q. Test	Alfred Binet
In Number Theory	Ramanujam
Incandescent Bulb	Edison
Induction Coil	Rohm Korff
Induction of Electric Current	Faraday
Insulin	F. Banting
Laughing Gas	Priestley
Law of Electrolysis	Faraday
Law of Gases	Gay Lussac
Laws of Electrical Resistance	Ohm
Laws of Gravitation	Newton
Laws of Heredity	Gregory Mandel
Laws of Inheritance	Gregory Mendel
Laws of Motion	Newton
Laws of Multiple Proportion	Dalton
Laws of Natural Selections	Darwin
Logarithms	John Napier

Machine Gun	Dr. Richard Gatling
Malarial Parasite	Ronald Ross
Match (safety)	J.E. Lurdstrom
Mathematical Astro-physics	Chandrasekhar
Mathematical Genius	Carl Gauss (Karl Friedrich Gauss)
Mauve Dye	Perkin
Measurement of Electrical Energy	Joule, James Prescoft
Mechanical Equivalent of Heat	Joules
Mercury Thermometer	Fahrenheit
Meson	Hideki Yakawa
Microphone	Johann Phillip Reis, Alexander Graham Bell, Elisha Gray, Amos E. Dolbear, and Thomas Edison
Microscopic Anatomy	Marcello Malpighi
Lift	E.g., Otis
Lift (Elevators)	Otis
Lightning Conductor	Benjamin Franklin
Line of Demarcation (Ship)	Plimsoll
Liquid Oxygen	Dewar
Locomotive	Richard Trevithick
Logarithmic Tables	John Napier
Motor Car (Petrol)	Karl Butler
Movie Projector	Thomas Alva Edison
Neon Gas	Ramsay, Travers
Neon Lamp	G. Claude
Neurophysiology	Charles Sherrington
Neutron	Chadwick
New Anatomy	Andreas Vesalius

CHEMISTRY

Matter and its states

- It exists in five states viz, solid, liquid, gas, plasma, Bose-Einstein condensate, out of which the former three are commonly seen.
- Anything that occupies space, possesses mass and can be felt by any one or more of our senses is called **matter**.

States of Matter

Solid State

A solid possesses definite shape and definite volume which means that it cannot be compressed on applying pressure.

Liquid State

A liquid possesses definite volume but no definite shape.

Gases

- These have neither definite volume nor definite shape.
- Solid, liquid and gases are inter-convertible by changing the conditions of temperature and pressure.
- **Fluorescent tube** contains helium (He) gas and neon sign bulb contains neon (Ne) gas.

Bose-Einstein condensate

- In 1924–25, Satyendra Nath Bose and Albert Einstein gave the information about Bose-Einstein condensate.
- It is a state of matter of a lower density gas of boson cooled up to temperature which is very close to absolute zero or –273.15°C. Infact, it is a fifth state of matter.
- **Pure substances:** A single substance (or matter) which cannot be separated into other kinds of matter by any physical process is called pure substance.

Elements

- They contain only single type of atoms.
- Elements which are liquid at room temperature are mercury (Hg) and bromine (Br_2).
- Examples (of elements) are diamond, graphite, sulphur (S_8), phosphorus (P_4), ozone (O_3), oxygen (O_2), etc.
- Elements have the following order of abundance in earth crust, Oxygen > silicon > aluminium (metal) > iron > calcium.

➢ Elements have the following order of abundance in human body: Oxygen > carbon > hydrogen > nitrogen.

Extraction Process for Various Elements

Frasch process	Sulphur
Acheson process	Graphite
Hall Herault	Aluminium
Ostwald process	Nitric acid
Bayer process	Extraction of aluminium from ore
Bessemer process	Steel from molten pig iron
Patio process	Silver
Dow process	Bromine
Pidgeion process	Magnesium
Fischer Tropsch process	Gasoline
Azeotropic distillation	Absolute alcohol

Metals

Metals are solids (exception mercury which is liquid at room temperature) are normally hard. They have lustre, high MP and BP and also with increase in temperature due to vibration of positive ions at their Lattice points.

Non-metals

Non-metals are the elements with properties opposite to those of the metals. They are found in all states of matter. They do not possess lustre (exception is iodine). They are poor conductors of electricity (exception is graphite) and they are not malleable and ductile.

Metalloids

Metalloids are the elements which have common properties of both metals and non-metals.

Compounds

Compounds are pure substances that are composed of two or more different elements in fixed proportion by mass.

➢ These contain more than one kind of atom.

➢ Their examples are silica (SiO_2), water (H_2O), sugar ($C_{12}H_{22}O_{11}$), salt (NaCl), etc.

Organic Compounds

The compounds obtained from living sources are called organic compounds. **Examples** are carbohyrates, proteins, oils, fats, etc.

Inorganic Compounds

The compounds obtained from non-living sources such as rocks and minerals are called inorganic compounds. **Examples** are common salt, marble, washing soda, etc.

Mixtures

A material obtained by mixing two or more substances in any indefinite proportion is called a mixture. **Examples** are milk, sea water, petrol, paint, glass, cement, wood, etc.

(a) Homogeneous Mixture

A mixture is said to be homogeneous if it does have a uniform composition throughout.

Example: Salt-solution, sugar solution, etc.

(b) Heterogeneous Mixture

A mixture is said to be heterogeneous if it does not have a uniform composition throughout and has visible boundaries of separation between the various constituents.

Example: A mixture of sulphur and sand, a mixture of iron fillings and sand, etc.

Separation of mixtures

Sublimation

In this process, a solid substance passes direct into its vapours on application of heat. The vapours when cooled, give back the original substance.

Filtration

This is a process for quick and complete removal of suspended solid particles from a liquid, by passing the suspension through a filter paper.

Evaporation

If a solution of solid substance in a liquid is heated, the liquid gets converted into its vapours and slowly goes off completely. This process is called evaporation.

Crystallisation

This method is mostly used for separation and purification of solid substances. In this process, the impure solid or mixture is heated with suitable solvent to its boiling point and the hot solution is filtered. The clear filtrate is cooled slowly to room temperature. When pure solid crystallises out, this is separated by filtration and dried.

Distillation

It is a process of converting a liquid into its vapour by heating and then condensing the vapour again into the same liquid by cooling. Thus, distillation involves vapourisation and condensation both.

(A) Vacuum Distillation

- It is also known as distillation under reduced pressures.

(B) Steam Distillation

- It is used to separate a steam volatile compound from non-volatile or non-steam volatile compounds.

(C) Fractional Distillation

- This process is similar to the distillation process except that a fractionating column is used to separate two or more volatile liquids which have different boiling points.

Concept of Change in State

(a) **Melting Point:** The temperature at which solid and the liquid forms of the substance exist at equilibrium or both forms have same vapour pressure is called melting point.

(b) **Boiling Point:** The temperature at which the vapour pressure of a liquid becomes equal to the atmospheric pressure is called boiling point.

(c) **Freezing Point:** The temperature at which a substance is changed from liquid state to solid state is called freezing point.

(d) **Vapour Pressure:** The pressure exerted by the vapours of liquid in equilibrium with liquid at a given temperature is called vapour pressure. Vapour pressure depends on (i) its nature and (ii) temperature.

Higher the vapour pressure, lesser will be the magnitude of intermolecular forces present in molecules. Vapour pressure of a liquid increases with increase in temperature.

Atomic Structure

Atom

The smallest particle of an element is called an atom. The atom of the hydrogen is the smallest and lightest.

Characteristics of Atoms

Atomic Number (Z)

- It is equal to the number of protons.
- It is equal to the number of electrons in netural atom.

Mass Number (A)

- It is equal to the sum of number of protons and number of neutrons.
- It is written as a superscript to the right of the symbol of the atom e.g., C^{12} here 12 is the mass number of carbon (C).

Molecule

A molecule is the smallest particle of a compound that can have a stable and independent existence.

Mole

A mole is a collection of 6.023×10^{23} particles.

Avogadro's Number

The number 6.023×10^{23} is called Avogadro's number.

Atomic Mass

It is the ratio of mass of one atom of the element to the part of the mass of one atom of Carbon-12.

Molecular Mass

It indicates how many times one molecule of a substance is heavier in comparison to the mass of the atom of Carbon-12.

Electron

i. Electron had been discovered by J.J. Thomson.
ii. The name of electron was given by Stoney.
iii. An electron was obtained from Cathode rays experiment.

- Its antiparticle is positron.
- It has mass 9.1×10^{-19} kg or 0.00054 u.
- It has charge -1.6×10^{-19} C (by Millikan oil drop experiment).

Proton

i. A proton had been discovered by Goldstein.
ii. A proton was named by Rutherford.
iii. A proton was obtained from anode rays experiment.

- It is positively charged.
- It is present in the nucleus.
- It has charge $+1.6 \times 10^{-19}$ C and mass 1.672×10^{-27} kg or 1.00727 u.

Neutron

i. A neutron had been discovered by James Chadwick.
ii. Charge on neutron is zero.
iii. A neutron was obtained from radioactivity phenomenon.

- It has zero charge and mass 1.674×10^{-17} kg or 1.00867 u.
- It is present inside the nucleus. Its antiparticle is antineutrino.

Atomic number (Z): The number of proton or electron in an atom of the element is called atomic number. It is denoted by **Z**.

Proton, Neutron and Electron Data

Particle	Relative Charge	Relative/C	Charge/kgs	Mass
Protons	1	+1	$+1.6\times10^{-19}$	$1.67\times10\times^{-27}$
Neutrons	1	neutral	0	1.67×10^{-27}
Electrons	0.0005	–1	-1.6×10^{-19}	9.11×10^{-31}

Nucleus

- It contains protons and neutrons which are collectively called nucleons.
- **Mass number (A):** The sum of number of protons and neutrons in an atom of the elements is called mass number. It is denoted by **A**.
- **Isotopes:** These are atoms of the elements having the same atomic number but different mass number.
- Hydrogen (H-1) is the lightest isotope and lead-208 is the heaviest isotope (with mass 207.974).
- **Thomson's model of an atom:** According to Thomson, an atom is treated as sphere of radius 10^{-8} cm in which positively charged particles are uniformly distributed and negatively charged electrons are embedded through them. This is also called Plum-Pudding model of an atom or watermelon model of an atom.

Cathode Rays

- These rays were discovered by J.J. Thomson.
- These rays originate from cathode and travels in a straight line towards anode.

Anode Rays

- These rays were discovered by Goldstein (also called positive rays).
- These rays do not originate from anode.
- These are positively charged and have velocity less than cathode rays.
- **Hydrogen** is the only atom in which neutrons are not present.
- According to **de-Broglie**, all particles have wave nature.

Radioactivity

- It was discovered by **Henry Becquerel** but term radioactivity was given by **Madam Curie**. It is the process of spontaneous disintegration of nucleus and is measured by Geiger counter.
- It involves emission of α, β and γ rays/particles and has units Curie, Becquerel, Rutherford.

Alpha (α) Particle

- These are positively charged helium nuclei $(2He_4)^{2+}$.
- An α-emission reduces the atomic mass by 4 and atomic number by 2.

Beta (β) Particle

- These are negatively charged electrons $(^{-1}e_0)$.
- A β-emission increases the atomic number by one with no change in atomic mass.

Gamma (γ) Rays

- These are electromagnetic radiations and have very high penetrating power.
- Their emission increases does not affect the position of nuclei in the Periodic Table.

Nuclear Reactor

- It is a device that is used to produce electricity and permits a controlled chain nuclear fission.
- It contains fuels e.g., $_{92}U^{235}$, moderator (e.g., graphite and heavy water, D_2O) to slow down neutrons and control rods (made up of boron steel or cadmium) to absorb neutrons.
- It may also contain liquid sodium as coolant.

Half-Life Period

- It is the time in which a radioactive substance remains half of its original amount.

Uses of RadioIcsotopes

1. **Iodine-131** is employed to study the structure and activity of thyroid gland.
2. **Iodine-123** is used in external radiation therapy for the treatment of cancer.
3. **Cobalt-60** is used in external radiation therapy for the treatment of cancer.
4. **Sodium-24** is injected along with salt solution to trace the flow of blood.
5. **Phosphorus-32** is used for leukemia therapy.
6. **Carbon-14** is used to study the kinetics of photosynthesis.

Radiocarbon Dating

- It is used in determining the age of carbon bearing materials such as wood, animal fossils, etc.

Uranium Dating

- It is used to determine the age of earth, minerals and rocks.

Periodic Classification of Elements

Father of Periodic Table is **Mendeleev**.

Periodic Table

- It is a tabular display of the chemical elements, organised on the basis of their properties.

Mendeleev's Periodic Table (1869)

- It is based upon the Mendeleev's periodic law, which states, "Properties of the elements are the periodic function of their atomic masses."

Modern Periodic Law: Modern periodic law was given by Moseley.

According to Moseley: "The physical and chemical properties of the elements are the periodic function of their atomic numbers."

Modern Periodic Table

It is just graphical representation of Aufbau principle. It is based on the electronic configuration of elements and contains 118 elements.

Modern periodic table is classified as:

i. *s*-block; ii. *p*-block; iii. *d*-block; iv. *f*-block.

S-Block

- It contains group 1 and 2, i.e., hydrogen and alkali metals (Li, Na, K, Rb, Cs, Fr) and alkatine earth metals (Be, Mg, Ca, Sr, Ba, Ra). General electronic configuration of these elements is ns^{0-2}.
- These elements are soft metals, electropositive.

P-Block

- It comprises the last six groups (13–18).
- General electronic configuration of this block elements is $ns^2\ np^{1-6}$.
- It is only block which contain metals, non-metals and metalloids.

D-Block

- It comprises 10 groups (3 to 12). These elements are called transition elements.
- General electronic configuration of d-block elements is $(n-1)d^{1-10}\ ns^{1-2}$.
- Hg, Zn, Cu, Sc etc. are d-block elements but not the transtion elements.

F-Block

- There are two series in this block 4 F and 5F series. 4F series elements are called lanthanides and 5F series elements are called actinides.
- General electronic configuration of this block elements is $(n-2)F^{1-14}\ (n-1)\ d^{1-10}\ ns^{1-2}$.

Chemical Bonding

The force that holds together the different atoms in a molecule is called chemical bond.

Ions

- These are of two types: cations and anions. **Cations** are formed by the loss of electrons and carry positive charge. **Anions** are formed by the gain of electrons and carry negative charge.

Ionic bond or (Electrovalent bond)

A bond formed by the complete transfer of ions or more electrons from one atom to other atom is called ionic bond.

Covalent bond

A bond formed between two same or different atoms by mutual contribution and sharing of electrons is called covalent bond.

Co-ordinate bond (or Dative bond): Co-ordinate bond is a special type of covalent bond in which one atom donates electrons of other atom. The bonding between donor to acceptor atom is called **co-ordinate bond.**

Valency

- It is the number of electrons taking part in bonding (i.e., bond formation).

Chemical Reaction

- The process in which substances (reactants) react to form new compunds (products) is known as chemical reaction.

Types of Reactions

Decomposition reactions: In these reactions, compound either of its own or upon heating decomposes to give two or more components out of which at least one is in the elemental state.

$$2\ KClO_3 \xrightarrow{\Delta} 2KCl + 3O_2$$

Potassium Chlorate → Potassium Chloride + Oxygen

Addition reactions: In such reactions, two or more substances combine to give a single substance.

Substitution reactions: In such reactions, an atom or a group of atoms of a molecule is replaced by another atom or group of atoms.

Combination reactions: In combination reactions, compounds are formed as a result of the chemical combination of two or more elements.

$$CaO + H_2O \longrightarrow Ca(OH)_2$$

Calcium Oxide + Water → Calcium Hydroxide

Displacement reactions: In these reactions, an atom/ion present in a compound gets replaced by an atom/ion of another element.

$$CuSO_4 + Fe \longrightarrow FeSO_4 + Cu$$

Copper Sulphate → Ferrous Sulphate

Disproportionation reactions: The chemical reaction in which only one substance is oxidised as well as reduced simultaneously is called disproportionation reaction.

Dissociation reactions: These are those reversible reactions in which a molecule dissociates into two or more simple molecules.

$2HI \rightleftharpoons H_2 + I_2$

Hydrogen iodide — Hydrogen — Iodine

Catalysis

- It was discovered by Berzelius.
- It is a term used for the reactions/processes which occur in the presence of certain substances that increase the rate of the reaction without being consumed. Such substances are called **catalysts**.

Uses of Catalysts

S. No.	Process	Catalyst
1.	Manufacture of Ghee from vegetable oils	Nickel
2.	Conversion of milk into curd	Lactase
3.	Decon's process for manufacture of chlorine	Cupric Chloride
4.	Conversion of sucrose into glucose and fructose	Invertase enzyme
5.	Contact process for manufacture of sulphuric acid	Pt Powder
6.	Conversion of proteins into peptide	Pepsin enzyme
7.	Conversion of glucose into ethyl alcohol	Zymase enzyme
8.	Formation of vinegar from cane sugar	Mesoderm acetate
9.	Conversion of starch into maltose	Diastase enzyme

Acids, Bases and Salts

Acid

An acid is a substance which

i. Is sour to taste.
ii. Turns blue litmus paper into red.
iii. Contains replaceable hydrogen.
iv. Gives hydrogen ion (H^+) in aqueous solution.
v. Can donate a proton.
vi. Can accept an electron.

Basicity of an acid: The number of removable hydrogen ions from an acid is called basicity of that acid.

Uses of HCl

i. Used as bathroom cleaner.
ii. As a pickling agent before galvanization.
iii. In the tanning of leather.
iv. In the dying and textile industry.
v. In the manufacture of gelatin from bones.

Uses of HNO_3

i. In the manufacture of explosives like TNT (Trinitrotoluene), TNB (Trinitrobenzene), Picric acid (Trinitrophenol), etc.
ii. Found in rain water (first shower).
iii. In the manufacture of rayon.

Uses of Sulphuric acid (H_2SO_4)

i. In lead storage battery.
ii. In the manufacturing of HCl.
iii. In the manufacturing of Alum.
iv. In the manufacturing of fertilisers, drugs, detergents and explosives.

Use of Boric Acid: It is used as an antiseptic.

Uses of Phosphoric Acid

i. Its calcium salt makes our bones.
ii. It forms phosphatic fertilisers.

Use of Ascorbic Acid: Source of vitamin C.

Use of Citric Acid: Flavouring agent and food preservative.

Use of Acetic Acid: Flavouring agent and food preservative.

Uses of Tartaric acid

i. Souring agent for pickles.
ii. A component of baking powder (sodium bicarbonate + tartaric acid).

Bases

A Base is a substance which:

i. Is bitter in taste.
ii. Turns red litmus paper into blue.
iii. Gives hydroxyl ions (OH^-) in aqueous solution.
iv. Can accept proton.
v. Can donate electrons.

- Oxides and hydroxides of metals are bases.
- Water soluble bases are called alkali.
- All alkalies are bases but all bases are not alkalies because all bases not soluble in water.

Acidity of a base: The number of removable hydroxyl (OH^-) ions from a base is called acidity of a base.

The pH scale: pH of a solution is the negative logarithm of the concentration of hydrogen ions on mole per litre.

Indicators

- These are the substances which give different colours in acid and base solution.

pH Value

- It is a measure of acidity or basicity of a solution.
- It is defined as the negative logarithm of the concentration in (mol/L) of hydrogen ions which it contains.
- It is seven for neutral solution, greater than seven for basic solution and less than seven for acidic solution.

Salts

- These are the product of neutralisation reaction between an acid and a base.

Washing Soda

- It is chemically sodium carbonate decahydrate ($Na_2CO_3.10H_2O$) and is used in glass, soap and paper industries and for removing permanent hardness of water.

Baking Soda

- It is sodium hydrogen carbonate ($NaHCO_3$). It is a mild non-corrosive base.
- When mixed with a mild edible acid such as tartaric acid it is called baking powder and is used to make bread or cake soft and spongy.

- It is used as mild antiseptic for skin infections, in soda-acids and as fire extinguishers.

Bleaching Powder

- It is chemically Ca (OCl)Cl or $CaOCl_2$.
- It is used for disinfecting drinking water.

Plaster of Paris

- It is chemically calcium sulphate hemihydrate.
- It is used to plaster fractured bones, for making toys, materials for decoration and for making surfaces smooth.

Copper Sulphate

- Copper sulphate when anhydrous, is white and when associated with water of crystallisation (i.e. $CuSO_4 . 5H_2O$), is blue, so it is called **blue vitriol**. It is used to test the presence of water.

Lime

- It is chemically calcium oxide and also called quicklime.
- It is used in the manufacture of glass, cement, etc. and for drying ammonia and alcohol.

Potassium Nitrate

- It is used as fertilizer in gun powder in matchsticks, etc.
- Ant or bee sting contains methanoic or **formic acid**.

Behaviour of Gases

Boyle's Law

At constant temperature, the volume of a definite mass of a gas is inversely proportional to pressure.

Charles' Law

- At constant pressure volume of a fixed mass of a gas is directly proportional to its absolute temperature.
- **Applications of Charles' Law**: Bursting of hydrogen balloon, making of chapatti.

Gay-Lussac's Law

At constant volume, the pressure of given mass of a gas is directly proportional to the temperature in Kelvin.

The Combined Gas Law or Ideal Gas Equation

- It is a gas law which combines Charles law, Boyle's law and Gay-Lussac's law.

Avogadro's Gas Law

At constant temperature and pressure the volume of a gas is directly proportional to the number of molecules.

Ideal Gas Equation

$PV = nRT$ is called ideal gas equation, where

P = Pressure
V = Volume
n = Number of mole
T = Temperature in Kelvin.

Diffusion of gases: The process of intermixing of gases irrespective of the density relationship and without the effect of external agency is called diffusion of gases.

Graham's Law of Diffusion

- According to this law, "the rate of diffusion of a gas is inversely proportional to the square root of its density."

Ideal and Real Gases

- Ideal gases follow gas laws in all conditions of temperature and pressure.
- **Critical temperature** is the temperature above which a gas cannot be liquefied.
- **Dalton's law of partial pressure:** It states that, if two or more gases which do not react chemically are enclosed in a vessel, the total pressure, of all gases of the gaseous mixture is equal to the sum of the partial pressures of all gases which exert pressure when enclosed separately in the same vessel at constant temperature.

Carbon and its Compounds

Allotropy

The substances which have same chemical properties, but different physical properties are called allotropes and this property is called allotropy.

Example: Allotropes of Carbon are diamond, graphite and charcoal.

Diamond

i. It is the purest form of carbon.
ii. It is hardest natural known substance.
iii. It is transparent and its specific gravity is 3.52.
iv. It is a bad conductor of electricity and heat.
v. It has very high refractive index of 2.415.
vi. It is chemically inert and on heating above 15000°C, it gets transformed into graphite.
vii. It has high MP and density.
viii. Black diamond called **Carbonado** contains traces of graphite.

Graphite (Plumbago or Black Lead)

i. It is soft, greasy, dark grayish colored crystalline solid.
ii. It is good conductor of heat and electricity.
iii. It is chemically more reactive than diamond.
iv. Its layer structure is headed by weak van der Waal's forces.

Fullerenes

- It (C60) looks like a soccer ball (or bucky-ball).

Graphene

- Graphene is an allotrope of carbon.

Carbon Monoxide (CO)

- It is formed by incomplete combustion. It is a colourless, odourless gas.

Organic Compounds

- These are the compounds of mainly carbon and hydrogen or compounds of carbon and hydrogen with other elements like phosphorus, oxygen, nitrogen, sulphur, halogens, etc.
- Urea is the first synthesised organic compound (by Wöhler).
- **Acetic acid** was the first organic compound synthesised in the laboratory from its elements.

Hydrocarbons

Compounds made of carbon and hydrogen atoms only, are called hydrocarbons. The natural source of hydrocarbons is petroleum.

1. **Saturated hydrocarbons:** The hydrocarbons in which carbon atoms are singly bonded are called saturated hydrocarbons. Saturated hydrocarbons are also called alkanes or paraffins.
   General formula of alkane $-C_nH_{2n+2}$.
2. **Unsaturated hydrocarbons:** The hydrocarbons in which carbon atoms are either doubly or triply bonded are called unsaturated hydrocarbons. Doubly bonded (carbon atoms) hydrocarbons are called alkenes. The general formula of alkene is C_nH_{2n}.

Triply-bonded carbon: Hydrocarbons containing at lease one carbon–carbon triple bond between two carbon atoms are called alkynes. The general formula of alkynes is C_nH_{2n-2}.

Aromatic Hydrocarbons

These are homocyclic compounds which contain at least one benzene ring in which carbon atoms are linked to one another by alternate single and double bonds.

Isomerism: Two or more compounds having same molecular formula but different physical and chemical properties are called isomers and this phenomenon is called isomerism.

Polymerisation: The simple molecules which combine to form a macro molecule called polymer. The process by which the simple molecules (monomers) are converted into polymer is called polymerisation.

Natural occurring polymers are protein, nucleic acid, cellulose, starch, etc.

Uses of Some Important Organic Compounds

- **Methane (CH_4)** is used to manufacture printer ink, methyl alcohol and to obtain light and energy.
- **Ethylene (C_2H_4)** is used to prepare mustard gas (war gas) and for ripening of fruits.
- **Glycol ($C_2H_6O_2$)** is used as an antifreeze mixture in car radiator and to prevent the freezing of fuel in spacecrafts.
- **Acetylene (C_2H_2)** is used to generate light, weld metals as oxy-acetylene flame and to prepare synthetic rubber (neoprene).
- **Methyl Alcohol (CH_3OH)** is used as a fuel with petrol, used to synthesise varnish and polish, used to denature ethanol.
- **Chloroform ($CHCl_3$)** is used as an anesthetic and to preserve substances obtained from plants and animals. It converts into poisonous phosgene ($COCl_2$), when exposed to sunlight. So, it is kept in dark bottles.
- **Glycerin ($C_3H_8O_3$)** is used as a preservative for fruits and juices, in leather industry and in coagulation of rubber.
- **Acetic acid (CH_3COOH)** is used in vinegar, medicines, and as a solvent.
- **Oxalic acid ($C_2H_2O_4$)** is used in printing of clothes, in photography and in the synthesis of coal tar.
- **Glucose ($C_6H_{12}O_6$)** is used for the synthesis of alcohol and as a preservative for fruit juice.
- **Benzene (C_6H_6)** is used as a solvent for oil fat and in drycleaning. Sodium benzoate is a food preservative.
- **Toluene ($C_6H_5CH_3$)** is used to synthesis explosive TNT, for drycleaning and for the synthesis of medicines like chloramine.
- **Phenol (C_6H_5OH)** is used to synthesis explosive, 2,4,6-trinitrophenol (picric acid) and bakelite.
- **Ethyl Alcohol (C_2H_5OH)** is used for drinking, in medicine to prepare tincture and as insecticide, and as a fuel with petrol.

Fuels

A substance that can supply energy either alone or by reacting with another substance is known as fuel. Heat produced by fuel is measured in Calories. An ideal fuel should:

i. Have high calorific value.
ii. Be cheap and easily available.
iii. Be easily stored and transport.
iv. Be regulated and controlled.
v. Have low ignition temperature.

The quantity of fuel is expressed in the form of calorific value.

Calorific Value

- It is defined as the heat obtained when 1 g of a fuel is burned in excess of oxygen and is expressed in kcal/g.
- **Hydrogen** is the fuel of future.
- Alcohol, when mixed with petrol, is called power alcohol. It is an alternative source of energy.
- For the **combustion of substance**, its ignition temperature should be low.

Flame

- It is the hot part of fire and has three parts:

1. **Innermost region**
   - It is black because of the presence of unburned carbon particles.
   - It has the lowest temperature.
2. **Middle region**
   - It is yellow luminous due to partial combustion of fuel.
3. **Outermost Region**
   - It is blue (non-luminous) due to complete combustion of fuel.
   - It is the hottest part of flame.

Metallurgy

The process of extracting metal in pure form from its ore is known as metallurgy.

Metals: These are the elements which are hard, lustrous, ductile, malleable, sonorous and conductor of heat and electricity in their solid as well as molten state. These evolve hydrogen gas when react with water and acids. Mercury (metal) is liquid at room temperature. Ti is called strategic metal.

Minerals: The compound of a metal found in nature is called a mineral.

Ores: Those minerals from which metal can be economically and easily extracted are called ores.

All ores are minerals but all minerals are not ores.

Gangue (or matrix): The ore is generally associated with earthy impurities like sand, rocks and limestone known as gangue or matrix.

Flux: A substance added to ore to remove impurities is called flux. There are two types of flux–(i) acidic flux, (ii) basic flux.

Slag: Combination of gangue with flux in ores forms a fusible material which is called slag.

Concentration: The process of removal of gangue from the ore is known as concentration of ore.

Calcination: It is the process of heating the concentrated ore in absence or in limited supply of air, below its melting point.

Roasting: Roasting is a process in which ore is heated usually in the presence of air, at temperatures below its melting point.

Smelting: The reduction of oxide ore with carbon at high temperature is known as smelting.

Corrosion

- It is the process of oxidative deterioration of a metal surface by the action of environment to form unwanted corrosion.
- Corrosion of iron is called rusting.
- It is prevented by the following methods:
  - By electroplating
  - By surface coating
  - By alloying
  - By galvanisation of iron

Alloys

- These are mixtures of two metals or a metal and a non-metal.

S. No.	Alloys	Constituents
1.	Brass	Copper (80%) & Zinc (20%)
2.	Bronze	Copper (90%) & Tin (1%)
3.	German Silver	Copper (60%), Zinc (20%) & Nickel (20%)
4.	Duralumin	Aluminium & Copper
5.	Alnico	Aluminium, Nickel, Cobalt & Iron
6.	Magnalium	Aluminium (95%) & Magnesium (5%)
7.	Babbitt Metal	Tin, Antimony, Copper & Lead. Used in ball bearings to reduce friction.
8.	Invar	Iron & Nickel. Used in precision instruments
9.	Bell metal	Copper & tin
10.	Gun Metal	Copper, Tin & Zinc
11.	Monel Metal	Nickel (67%), Copper & Iron
12.	Pewter	Tin (80-90%), Copper & Lead
13.	Solder	Tin, Lead & Antimony

Compounds of Metals and Non-Metals and Their Uses

1. **Ferrous sulphate** ($FeSO_4$). $4H_2O$: In dye industry, and Mohr's salt.
2. **Iodine** (I_2): (i) As antiseptic, (ii) In making tincture of iodine.
3. **Bromine** (Br_2): (i) In dye industry (ii) As a laboratory reagent.
4. **Chlorine** (Cl_2): In the formation of (i) Mustard gas (ii) Bleaching.
5. **Sulphuric acid** (H_2SO_4): (i) As a reagent (ii) In purification of petroleum (iii) In lead storage battery.
6. **Sulphur** (S): Antiseptics, vulcanization of rubber, gun powder, medicine.
7. **Phosphorus (P)** : (i) Red Phosphorus refrigerant, in match industry, etc. (ii) White Phosphorus–Rat killing Medicine.
8. **Carbon dioxide** (CO_2): Soda water, Fire extinguisher.
9. **Graphite:** As electrodes.
10. **Alum** [$K_2SO_4Al_2$ $(SO_4)_3.H_2O$]: (i) Purification of water (ii) Leather industry.
11. **Mercuric Chloride** ($HgCl_2$): Calomel, Insecticides (Corrosive sublimate).
12. **Mercuric oxide (HgO):** Ointment, poison.
13. **Zinc Sulphide (ZnS):** White pigment.
14. **Zinc Sulphate (White vitriol)** ($ZnSO_4{:}7H_2O$): Lithopone, Eye ointment.
15. **Zinc Chloride ($ZnCl_2$):** Textile industry.
16. **Zinc oxide (ZnO):** Ointment.
17. **Plaster of Paris** [$(CaSO_4)_2$. $2H_2$/ $CaSO_4$½H_2O)]: Statue, Surgery.
18. **Calcium sulphate ($CaSO_4$. $2H_2O$):** Cement industry.
19. **Calcium carbonate ($CaCO_3$):** Lime and toothpaste..
20. **Cupric oxide (CuO):** Blue and green glass, purification of petroleum.
21. **Cuprous Oxide (Cu_2O):** Red Glass, pesticides.
22. **Copper (Cu):** Electrical wire.
23. **Sodium nitrate ($NaNO_3$):** Fertilizer.
24. **Sodium Sulphate (Glauber's salt) ($Na_2SO_4.10H_2O$):** Medicine, cheap glass.
25. **Sodium bicarbonate (Baking soda) ($NaHCO_3$):** Fire extinguisher, bakery, reagent.
26. **Sodium Carbonate (Washing soda):** (i) Glass industry, (ii) Paper industry, (iii) Removal of permanent hardness of water, (iv) Washing.
27. **Heavy Water (D_2O):** Nuclear reactor.
28. **Liquid Hydrogen:** Rocket fuel.

Elements/Compounds and Their Uses

Element/Compound	Uses
Xenon	High-speed photographic tubes. Electric valves and T.V. tubes
Krypton	Incandescent bulb. Airfield lights because of characteristic red colour.
Lithium	Deoxidizer and to remove unwanted gases during the manufacture of metals.
Beryllium X-ray	(Transparent) window. Moderator in nuclear reactions around the core.
Neon	Neon lights. Cryogenics
Hopsalite	Mixture of oxides of manganese, cobalt, copper and silver-Antipollution
Ammonia	Refrigerant, fertilisers
Yttrium	Used in TVs to produce red colour
Bismuth	Mixed with iron to make it malleable
Sodium	Street lamp

Gadolinium	CDs. Aluminium is sometimes used to coat the disc
Cesium	Atomic clocks
Tellurium	Tint glass (one-way visibility used in cars)
Technetium	Superconductor at–262 degree Celsius
Paraformaldehyde	Common disinfectant and contraceptives
Potassium Dichromate	Used in breath analyser for detecting alcohol. Safe limit is 0.1%.

Non-Metal

- In Modern Periodic Table, there are 24 non-metals.
- Electronegative elements are non-metals.
- Non-metals are bad conductors of heat and electricity except graphite, Bi and Ge are semi-conductors.
- Protium is the only one isotope in Periodic Table having zero neutrons.
- Deuterium oxide is known as heavy water and used in nuclear reactor as moderator.
- Liquid hydrogen is used as rocket fuel.
- Hydrogen is known as range element because it may kept in group I and group VII A.
- These may be solid, liquid or gas (bromine is the only liquid non-metal).
- These are soft, non-lustrous, brittle, non-sonorous and non-conductor of heat and electricity.
- These form oxides with oxygen which are generally acidic.

Helium

- It is noble gas.
- It is used for filling balloons and other lighter aircraft.
- Helium (He), when mixed with O_2, is used by deep-sea divers for breathing and for respiratory patients.

Neon

- It is used in neon signs.

Argon

- It is used to generate inert atmosphere for welding and to fill incandescent light bulbs.

Xenon

- It is called stranger gas.

Water (H_2O)

Hard water–Less froth with soap.
Soft water–More froth with soap.

Oxygen

Ozone (O_3) is the allotrope of Oxygen.

Nitrogen

78% by volume in atmosphere, liquid nitrogen is used for refrigeration. Ammonia is an important compound of N_2 which is prepared by Haber's process.

Ammonia

- As refrigerant, in the manufacture of HNO_3.
- In fertilizer like urea, ammonium sulphate, etc.
- In the manufacture of Na_2CO_3 and $NaHCO_3$.
- In preparation of ammonium salt.
- In preparation of explosive.
- In preparation of artificial silk.
- Nitrogen fixation in leguminous plants.

Phosphorous

- An important constituent of animals and plants. It is present in bones and DNA.

Halogens

- **Fluorine** is used in the preparation of UF_6 and SF_6 for energy production and as dielectric constant, respectively.
- By using HF, chlorofluorocarbon compound and polytetrafluoroethylene can be synthesised.
- Chlorofluorocarbon is known as Freon and is used as refrigerant and aerosol.
- Non-stick utensils are made up of teflon.
- **Chlorine** is used to prepare PVC, insecticides herbicides, etc.
- **Bromine** is used in ethylene bromide synthesis which is mixed with leaded petrol.

Inert Gases

- They belong to 18th group of Periodic Table. For example, He, Ne, Ar, Kr, Xe, Rn.
- Except Rn, all inert gases are present in atmosphere.
- Argon is used in Arc. welding and electric bulbs.
- Helium is light and non-inflammable so, used in balloon, weather indicator, etc.
- Neon is used in discharge tube glow light.

Some Important Explosives

- **Dynamite:** It was discovered by Alfred Nobel in 1863. It is prepared by absorption of raw dust with nitro-glycerin. In modern dynamite, Sodium Nitrate is used in place of Nitro-glycerin.
- **Tri Nitro Phenol (TNP):** It is also known as picric acid.
- **R.D.X.** is highly explosive known as plasticiser in which aluminium powder is mixed to increase the temperature and the speed of fire.

Man-made substances

- **Fertilisers:** The substances added to the soil to make up the deficiency of essential elements are known as fertilisers, these are either natural or synthetic (chemical).
  Among the chemical fertilisers, the two important categories are:
- **Phosphate fertilisers:** The most abundant phosphate is rock phosphate [$3Ca_3(PO_4)_2$], which is mostly consumed by the fertiliser industry in the manufacture of 'superphosphate of lime', 'triple superphosphate' and 'altrophs'–a combined phosphatic and nitrogenous fertiliser.
  Nitrogenous Fertilizers: Plants need nitrogen for rapid growth and increase in their protein content. For this reason, nitrogenous fertilizers are of some more importance. The chief nitrogenous fertilizers are ammonium sulphate, calcium cyanamide, sodium nitrate, ammonium nitrate, urea, and ammonium phosphate.
- **Dyes:** Coloured substances used for colouring textiles, foodstuffs, silk, wool, etc. are called dyes.
- **Cement:** It is a complex material containing the silicates of calcium and aluminium. A paste of sand, cement and water is called mortar.

A mixture of stone chips (gravel), cement and water is known as concrete. Concrete with steel bars and wires is called reinforced concrete. It is used for constructing roads, bridges and pillars.

- **Glass:** It is an amorphous or transparent solid, also called **supercooled liquid**. It mainly contains silica (SiO_2).

Different kinds of glass are as follows:

1. **Soda or soft glass** is sodium calcium silicate used for making bottles, window panes, etc.
2. **Potash glass or hard glass** contains potassium. It is used for making chemical apparatus: beakers, flasks, funnel, etc.
3. **Crown glass** contains potassium oxide, barium oxide, boric oxide, and silica. It is used for optical apparatus.
4. **Flint glass** contains lead oxide and is used in optical instruments like lenses, prisms.
5. **Crook's glass** contains cesium oxide. It is used for spectacles as it absorbs UV rays.
6. **Jena glass** contains B_2O_3 and alumina. It is used for making laboratory bottles, for keeping acids and alkalies.
7. **Milky glass** is prepared by adding tin oxide, calcium phosphate or cryolite to the melt glass.
8. Glass laminates is made by fixing polymer sheets between layers of glass. It is used to make window and screens of cars, trains and aircraft. Specially manufactured glass laminates are used as bulletproof material.

   It has the following composition: calcium oxide (CaO) = 50–60%, silica (SiO_2) = 20–25%, alumina (Al_2O_3) = 5–10%; magnesium oxide (MgO) = 2–3%.

   It is manufactured from limestone and clay.

- **Paint:** A chemical that contains a pigment as a vehicle and a thinner.

White pigment: Zinc oxide, white lead and titanium dioxide. The pigment mixed with a vehicle, which is an oil like ***linseed* or *soyabean*** oil a ***polymer.*** A thinner is a solvent such as ***turpentine oil* or *kerosene.***

Luminous paints: Glow when exposed to light.

- **Soaps:** These are sodium and potassium salts of higher fatty acids.
- **Detergents:** These are sodium or potassium salts of long chain alkyl or aryl sulphonates or sulphates.
- These are also called **soapless soap**.
- **Antibiotic:** Medicinal compounds produced by moulds and bacteria, capable of destroying or preventing the growth of bacteria in animal systems.
- **Antibody:** Kinds of substances formed in the blood, tending to inhibit or destroy harmful bacteria, etc.
- **Antidote:** Medicine used against a poison.
- **Antigen:** Substance capable of stimulating formation of antibodies.
- **Antipyretics** are used to reduce body temperature during high fever, e.g., paracetamol, aspirin, phenacetin, analgin, and novalgin.
- **Tranquilizers** are used to treat stress, mild, and severe mental disease.
- **Antiseptic:** Prevent the growth of microorganisms or kill them but are not harmful to living tissues, e.g., dettol and savlon.
- **Analgesics:** Painkillers are called analgesics, e.g., aspirin, paracetamol and morphine.
- **Antimalarials** are used to treat malaria, e.g., chloroquin.
- **Sulphadrugs:** Alternatives of antibiotics, sulphanilamide, sulphadiazine sulphagunamidine.
- **Antacid:** Substances which remove the excess acid and raise the pH to appropriate level in scotch are called antacids.
- **Antacids** are used as a remedy for acidity.
- **Pesticides** are used to destroy the organisms that harm the crop.

These are of the following types.

1. **Insecticides,** e.g., DDT, aluminium phosphate, gammexane.
2. **Fungicide,** e.g., Bordeaux mixture.
3. **Herbicides,** e.g., benzepam, benzadox.
4. **Rodenticides,** e.g., aluminium phosphide.

- **Chloroform:** A sweetish, colourless liquid. It is used as a solvent and anaesthetic.
- **Saccharin:** A white crystalline solid which is 550 times sweeter than sugar, but does not have any food value. It is used by diabetic patients
- **DDT:** Dichlorodiphenyltricholoro ethane is a white powder used as an insecticide.

Propellants

Liquid propellants	Liquid hydrogen, liquid ammonia, hydrazine, nitromethane, methyl nitrate, hydrogen peroxide
Solid propellants	Polybutadiene, acrylic acid, nitroglycerine + nitrocellulose
Hybrid propellants	N_2O_4 + Acrylic rubber
	Dyes
Nitro dyes	Less important as the colours are not fast
Azo dyes	Azo (-N=N-) group is chromophore
Triphenylmethane dye	Malachite green
Direct dyes	Mautius yellow, Naphthol yellow, Congo red, etc.
Mordant dyes	Alizarin
Vat dyes	Indigo

BIOLOGY

Classification of Organisms

Classification means to categorise organisms into different groups.

1. Monera

It includes all prokaryotic organisms like bacteria, cynobacteria and archiobacteria.

2. Protista

This kingdom includes unicellular form usually found in parasitic and saprophytic forms. Euglena has both heterotrophic and autotrophic modes of nutrition.

3. Fungi

This kingdom includes non-green plants. It has saprophytic nutrition and growing on dead and decaying organic matter.

Example: Mushroom, Mucor, Albugo, etc.

4. Plantae

This kingdom includes all plants except some algae, diatoms, fungi and ember of monera and protista.

5. Animalia

Almost all animals come under this kingdom except protozoan.

Study of Cell

- **Cell:** The **Cell** is the basic structural and functional unit of all known living organisms. It is the smallest unit of life and is often called the building block of life.
- The largest known cells are unfertilized **ostrich egg** cells.
- The smallest cell is of **PPLO** (*Mycoplasma gallisepticum*).
- Human nerve cell is the **longest animal cell.**
- Largest unicellular plant is Acetabularia (10 cm) and animal is *Amoeba,* (1mm).
- The largest human cell is the **female ovum** and the smallest human cell is the **red blood cell.**
- **Robert Hooke** coined the term *cell.*
- The first living cell was discovered by **Leeuwenhoek.**
- The longest cell is *Neuron.*
- The biggest cell is egg of *Ostrich.*

Types of Cells

i. **Prokaryotic Cells:** These are primitive cells, lacking a nucleus and most of the other cell organelles.

ii. **Eukaryotic Cells:** These have nucleus and membrane bound cell organelles.

Difference Between Eukaryotic Cells and Prokaryotic Cells

Cell organelle	Eukaryotic	Prokaryotic
Nucleus	Present	Absent
Number of chromosomes	More than one	One–but not true chromosome: Plasmids
Cell Type	Usually multicellular	Usually unicellular (some cyanobacteria may be multicellular)
True Membrane-bound Nucleus	Present	Absent
Example	Animals and plants	Bacteria and archaea
Genetic Recombination	Meiosis and fusion of gametes	Partial, undirectional transfers, DNA
Lysosomes and peroxisomes	Present	Absent
Microtubules	Present	Absent or rare
Endoplasmic reticulum	Present	Absent
Mitochondria	Present	Absent
Cytoskeleton	Present	May be absent
DNA wrapping on proteins	Eukaryotes wrap their DNA around proteins called histones	Multiple proteins act together to fold and condense prokaryotic DNA. Folded DNA is then organized into a variety of conformations that are supercoiled and wound around tetramers of the HU protein.
Ribosomes	Larger	Smaller
Vesicles	Present	Present
Golgi apparatus	Present	Absent
Chloroplasts	Present (in plants)	Absent; chlorophyll scattered in the cytoplasm
Flagella	Microscopic in size; membrane bound; usually arranged as nine doublets surrounding two singlets	Submicroscopic in size, composed of only one fiber
Permeability of nuclear membrane	Selective	Not present
Plasma membrane with steroid	Yes	Usually no
Cell wall	Only in plant cells and fungi (chemically simpler)	Usually chemically complexed
Vacuoles	Present	Present
Cell size	10-100 μm	1-10 μm

Main Features of the Cell Theory

1. All organisms are composed of cell.
2. Each cell arises from pre-existing cell.
3. Every organism starts its life from single cell.

Parts of cell and their functions

1. **Cell wall:** In plant cell there is a rigid cell wall which is non-living and freely permeable. It is made up of cellulose and chitin. It provides shape and rigidity to the cell.
2. **Cell membrane:** It is also known as plasma membrane which form the outer covering of animal cell. In plant cell it is found within cell wall.
   Function: It regulates movement of molecules inside and outside of the cell.
3. **Protoplasm:** The whole fluid present inside plasma-membrane is protoplasm.
   (A) **Cytoplasm:** The fluid found outside the nuclear membrane.
   (B) **Nucleoplasm:** The fluid found inside the nuclear membrane.

Mitochondria

➢ It is a semi-autonomous organelle and called **powerhouse of the cell** because in it stepwise oxidation of fuel occurs which results in release of chemical energy. This energy is stored in the form of ATP.

Endoplasmic Reticulum

➢ These are hollow membranous system having ribosomes (thus called Rough ER) or no ribosomes (thus called Smooth ER). Rough Endoplasmic Reticulum is the site of protein synthesis, while Smooth Endoplasmic Reticulum is the site of synthesis of steroids and detoxification.

Golgi Apparatus

➢ Play important role in secretion, transportation and acrosome formation.

Plastid

Only found in plant cells.

(a) **Chloroplasts:** These are green pigment found in green planted involved in photosynthesis. So, it is known as *'Kitchen of the cell'*.
   Function: Chloroplast provides green colour to plant and take part photosynthesis.

(b) **Chromoplast** provides various colours to the plant.

(c) **Leucoplast** is colourless. It stores the food in the form of starch, lipid or protein.
   Functions:
   i. It helps in osmoregulation. It stores toxic metabolic water.
   ii. It controls all the activities of a cell. So, it is also known as the 'control-room' of a cell. Chromatin transmits hereditary characters from parents to their offspring.

The red colour of tomatoes is due to the presence of lycopene pigment, i.e., chromophore.

The colour of **carrot** is due to carotene.

Ribosomes

It is made up of ribonucleic acid (RNA).

Functions

i. Take part in protein synthesis.
ii. It helps in intracellular digestion. The enzyme found in lysosome may digest the entire cell. So it is also known as suicidal bag.
iii. Help in the formation of spindle fibre during cell division.

Chromosome

➢ Chromosome is thread-like structure, found in the nucleus. Bead-like structure found on chromosome is called **genes,** which are made up of DNA and are the carrier of genetic information from generation-to-generation. In some viruses, RNA is the genetic material called **retrovirus.**

➢ Eukaryotic cells possess many chromosomes.

Organism	Number of pairs of chromosomes
Dog	39 = 78
Human	23 = 46
Monkey	21 = 42
Onion	8 = 16

Difference between plant and animal cell

Plant cell	Animal cell
It has cell wall.	Cell wall is usually absent.
Plastids are found.	Plastids are usually absent.
A big vacuole is present.	Vacuole is absent or very small in size

Lysosomes

➢ These are sometimes called **suicidal bags of the cell.**

Centrosomes

➢ Participate in the formation of spindle during cell division and cilia.

Vacuoles

➢ These are non-living reservoirs, bounded by a membrane called **tonoplast.**

➢ It stores toxic metabolic waste and helps in osmoregulation.

Nucleus

➢ It was discovered by **Robert Brown.**

➢ Nucleus is rich in protein and RNA. Chromatin is the **controlling centre of a cell.**

Nucleic Acids

➢ These contain the genetic instructions used in the development and functioning of all known **living organisms.**

➢ These are of two types DNA and RNA.

Deoxyribonucleic Acid (DNA)

➢ It is a long polymer made from repeating units called **nucleotides.**

➢ Each nucleotide consists of a nucleoside and a phosphate group, joined together by ester bonds.

➢ It has four bases, e.g., adenine, guanine, cytosine and thymine.

➢ DNA was discovered by **James D Watson** and Francis Crick, who got Nobel Prize for this discovery.

DNA Synthesise RNA

☞ **Note: DNA:** DNA is mainly found in nucleus in small amount it is also found in mitochondria and chloroplast.

Gene: Gene is hereditary unit which is made by a segment of DNA found on the chromosome.

Ribonucleic Acid (RNA): RNA is single stranded nucleic acid made up to phosphate, ribose sugar and nitrogenous base uracil, adenine, guanine and cytosine. It is found in nucleus as well as cytoplasm.

Function: Synthesis of protein.

Comparison of DNA and RNA

Comparison	DNA	RNA
Name	Deoxyribonucleic acid	Ribonucleic acid
Function	Long-term storage of genetic information; transmission of genetic information to make other cells and new organisms.	Used to transfer the genetic code from the nucleus to the ribosomes to make proteins. RNA is used to transmit genetic information in some organisms and may have been the molecule used to store genetic blueprints in primitive organisms.
Structural Features	B-form double helix. DNA is a double-stranded molecule consisting of a long chain of nucleotides.	A-form helix. RNA usually is a single-strand helix consisting of shorter chains of nucleotides.
Composition of Bases and Sugars	Deoxyribose sugar Phosphate backbone Adenine, guanine, cytosine, thymine bases	Ribose sugar Phosphate backbone Adenine, guanine, cytosine, uracil bases
Propagation	DNA is self-replicating.	RNA is synthesized from DNA on an as-needed basis.
Base-pairing	AT (adenine-thymine) GC (guanine-cytosine)	AU (adenine-uracil) GC (guanine-cytosine)
Reactivity	The C-H bonds in DNA make it fairly stable, plus the body destroys enzymes that would attack DNA. The small grooves in the helix also serve as protection, providing minimal space for enzymes to attach.	The O-H bond in the ribose of RNA makes the molecule more reactive, compared with DNA. RNA is not stable under alkaline conditions, plus the large grooves in the molecule make it susceptible to enzyme attack. RNA is constantly produced, used, degraded, and recycled.
Ultraviolet Damage	DNA is susceptible to UV damage.	Compared with DNA, RNA is relatively resistant to UV damage.

Cell cycle

It is the sequence of events in which cell duplicates its genetic material, synthesises the other constituents of the cell and ultimately divide into two daughter cells.

Cell Division

The process in which cells increase in their number is called cell division.

(A) **Mitosis:** Mitosis cell division occurs in somatic cells which take part in growth, repair and development. In an unicellular organism, asexual reproduction takes place by this type of cell division.

(B) **Meiosis:** Meiosis cell division occurs in a reproductive cell. This type of division takes place during the formation of haploid gamete, i.e, over a sperm.

ZOOLOGY

Animal Tissue

i. **Epithelial Tissue:** Epithelial tissue cover the external surface of the body and internal free surface of many organs.
   Example: skin, intestine, gland.

ii. **Connective Tissue:** These tissues connect and bind different tissues and organs.
   Example: Adipose tissue found beneath the skin. Ligament is made up of fibrous connective tissue, cartilage, bone and blood.

☞ **Note:** Blood is only tissue which is found in the form of fluid.

iii. **Muscular Tissue:** This is also known as contractile tissue. All the muscles of the body are made up of this tissue.

(a) **Unstriped:** This muscle tissue is found on the walls of those parts which are not controlled by will.

(b) **Striped:** These muscles are found in the parts of the body that move voluntarily.

(c) **Cardiac:** These muscles are found only on the walls of the heart.

The largest muscle of the human body is Gluteus Maximus.

The smallest muscle of the human body is Stapedius.

iv. **Nervous Tissue:** This tissue is also called sensitive tissue.

Human Blood

- The quantity of blood in the human's body is 7% of the total weight.
- Blood is fluid connective tissue and composed of blood corpuscles, plasma and platelets.
- It is slightly alkaline in nature (pH 7.4).
- Its volume in an adult is 5.8 L.
- People who live at high altitudes have more blood than those who live in low regions. This extra blood supplies additional oxygen to body cells.
- During blood clotting fibrinogen changes into fibrin by thrombin which is obtained from thromboplastin in the presence of Ca^{2+}.
- Female contains half litre of blood less in comparison to male.

Blood Consists of Two Parts

(A) Plasma; and (B) Blood corpuscles.

(A) **Plasma:** This is the liquid part of blood. 60% of the blood is plasma. Its 90% part is water, 7% protein, 0.9% salt and 0.1% is glucose.

- **Function of plasma:** Transportation of digested food, hormones, excretory product, etc. from the body takes place through plasma.
- **Serum:** When Fibrinogen and protein is extracted out of plasma the remaining plasma is called serum.

(B) **Blood corpuscles:** This is the remaining 40% part of the blood.

i. **Red Blood Corpuscles (RBC):** Red Blood Corpuscles (RBC) in mammal is biconcave.
   - There is no nucleus in it. Exception–Camel and Lama. RBC is formed in Bone marrow.
   - Its life span is from 20 days to 120 days.
   - Its destruction takes place in liver and spleen. Therefore, liver is the grave of RBC.
   - It contains haemoglobin, in which haeme iron containing compound found and due to this the colour of blood is red.
   - The main function of RBC is to carry oxygen to all cells of the body bring back the carbon dioxide.

ii. **White Blood Corpuscles (WBC) or Leucocytes:**
   - Its formation takes place in Bone marrow, lymph node and sometimes in liver and spleen.
   - Its life span is from 1 to 2 days.
   - Nucleus is present in the White Blood Corpuscles.
   - Its main function is to protect the body from the disease. The ratio of RBC and WBC is 600 : 1.

iii. **Blood Platelets or Thrombocytes:** It is found only in the blood of human and other mammals.
   - There is no nucleus in it.
   - Its formation takes place in Bone marrow.
   - Its life span is from 3 to 5 days.
   - It dies in the Spleen.
   - Its main function is to help in clotting of blood.

Functions of Blood

i. To control the temperature of the body and to protect the body from diseases.
ii. Clotting of blood.
iii. Transportation of O_2, CO_2, digested food, conduction of hormones, etc.
iv. To help in establishing coordination among different parts.

➢ The main reason behind the difference in blood of human is the glycoprotein which is found in Red Blood Corpuscles called antigens. Antigens are of two types: Antigen A and Antigen B.

➢ On the basis of presence of Antigen or Glycoprotein, there are four group of blood in human:
   (a) That contains Antigen A–Blood Group A.
   (b) That contains Antigen B–Blood Group B.
   (c) That contains both the Antigens A and B–Blood Group AB.
   (d) That contains neither of the Antigens–Blood Group O.

An opposite type of protein is found in blood plasma. This is called antibody. This is also of two types–Antibody 'a' and Antibody 'b'.

Blood Transfusion: Antigen 'A' and antibody 'a', Antigen 'B' and antibody 'b' cannot live together. In case of so happened these get most sticky, such spoils the blood. This is called agglutination of blood.

Blood Group **O** is called **Universal Donor** because it does not contain any antigen.

Blood Group **AB** is called **Universal Receptor** because it does not contain any antibody.

If in the blood of people it is found, their blood is said to be Rh-positive and if in the blood of people it is not found, their blood is said to be Rh-negative.

At the time of blood transfusion, Rh-factor is also tested. Rh-positive is given to Rh-positive blood and Rh-negative is given to Rh-negative blood only.

Possible Combinations of Blood Groups

Male	Female	Blood group of Children not possible
A	A	B & AB
A	B	–
A	AB	O
A	O	B or AB
B	B	A, AB
B	AB	O
B	O	A, AB
AB	AB	O
AB	O	O, AB
O	O	A, B, AB

Blood Pressure (BP)

➢ The pressure created by the blood on the walls of the blood vessels due to the repeated pumping of heart is called **blood pressure**. It is measured by **sphygmomanometer.**

➢ Blood pressure in a normal person is 120/80 mm Hg.

➢ If a person has persistent high blood pressure then it is called hypertension and persistent high blood pressure is 150/90 mm Hg.

➢ **Hypotension** is condition of low blood pressure, *i.e.,* persistent 100/50 mm Hg.

➢ Electrocardiograph (ECG) is used to check proper working of heart.

System of the Human Body

Epidermis

➢ The top layer of skin made up of epithelial cells and does not contain blood vessels.

Dermis

➢ It gives elasticity to the integument, allowing stretching and conferring flexibility, while resisting distortions, wrinkling and sagging.

Hypodermis

➢ It is made up of adipose tissue.

Teeth

➢ With the help of teeth the food is chewed. Teeth are of four types
   i. Incisors
   ii. Canines
   iii. Premolars
   iv. Molars

➢ Hardest part in the body is tooth enamel.

Tongue

- Saliva, secreted by the salivary glands, is mixed with the chewed food by the tongue.
- Complete digestion process takes place in following four steps:
  - i. Ingestion of Food
  - ii. Digestion in Mouth.
  - iii. Digestion in Stomach.
  - iv. Digestion in Intestine.
- The food passes down through the oesophagus into stomach.
- Now food is mixed with gastric juice and hydrochloric acid which disinfect the food and creates acidic medium.
- Pepsin digests proteins and converts them into peptones.
- Renin coverts milk into curd.
- The digested food now is called chyme.
  1. **Ingestion:** Taking the food into the mouth is called ingestion.
  2. **Digestion:** Conversion of non-absorbable food into absorbable form. The digestion of the food is started in the mouth.
- Saliva is secreted by salivary gland in mouth in which two types of enzymes are found, ptyalin and maltase. They convert starch into simple sugar and make it digestible.
- From the mouth the food goes into stomach through foodpipe.
- No digestion takes place in foodpipe.

Digestion in Stomach

- The food lies approximately for four hours in the stomach.
- Hydrochloric acid secreted from the Oxyntic cells of the stomach kill all the bacteria coming with food and accelerate the reaction of enzymes.
- The enzymes in the gastric juice of stomach are–Pepsin and Renin.
- Pepsin breaks down the protein into peptones.
- Renin breaks down the caseinogen into casein.

Small Intestine

Digestion in Intestine

Food passes into ileum and mixes with intestinal juice, where:

- Maltase converts into glucose.
- Lactose converts into glucose and galactose.
- Sucrose converts into glucose and fructose.
- Trypsin digests the peptides into amino acids.
- Food now is called chyle.

The main organs participating in digestion:

Liver: This is the largest gland of the human body. Its weight is approximately 1.5–2 kilogram.

- Bile is secreted through liver only.
- Liver converts excess of amino acid into ammonia by deamination. The ammonia is further converted into urea by ornithine cycle. Urea comes out from body through kidney.
- Liver converts some quantity of protein into glucose during defecation of carbohydrate.
- Liver regulates the quantity of glucose in the blood.
- In case of decrease of fat in food liver converts some of the parts of carbohydrates into fat.
- The production of fibrinogen protein takes place by liver which helps in clotting of blood.
- The production of Heparin protein takes place in liver which prevent the clotting of blood inside the body.
- The liver reserves some quantity of iron, copper and vitamin.
- It helps in regulating the body temperature.
- Liver is an important clue in investigating a person's death that is been due to poison in food.

Gall Bladder: Gall bladder is a pear shaped sac, in which the bile coming out of liver is stored.

- Bile is a yellowish-green coloured alkaline liquid, whose pH value is 7.7.
- The quantity of water is 85% and the quantity of bile pigment is 12% in water.

The main functions of bile are as under:

- i. It makes the medium of food alkaline so that pancreatic juice can work.
- ii. It kills the harmful bacteria coming with food.
- iii. It emulsifies the fats.
- iv. It accelerates the bowel movement of intestine by which digestive juices in the food mix well.
- v. It is helpful in the absorption of vitamin K and other vitamins mixed in fats.

In case of obstruction in bile duct, liver cells stop taking bilirubin form. As a result, bilirubin spreads throughout the body. This is called jaundice.

Pancreas: This is the second largest gland of the human body. It acts simultaneously as endocrine and exocrine type of gland.

Islets of Langerhans: This is a part of the pancreas.

- **Insulin:** It is secreted by β-Cells of Islets of Langerhans which is a part of pancreas.
  It controls the process of making glycogen from glucose.
  Diabetes is caused due to the deficiency of insulin.
- Excessive flow of insulin causes Hypoglycemia in which one loses the producing capacity and vision deterioration.
  Glucagon: It re-converts the glycogen into glucose.

CIRCULATORY SYSTEM

The discovery of blood circulation was done by William Harvey.

Heart

It remains safe in the pericardial membrane.

Heart of the human is made up of four chambers.

- The chamber which receives the blood from body tissues is called **auricles** and the chambers of heart which pump blood to body tissues are called **ventricles.**
- There is a thin two layered sac around the heart known as **pericardium,** filled with a watery fluid called pericardial fluid, which allows frictionless movements of heart and protects it from mechanical shocks.
- The blood vessel: carrying the blood from the body towards the heart is called vein.
- In the vein there is impure blood i.e. carbon dioxide mixed blood with the exception is pulmonary vein, which always carry pure blood.

- Pulmonary vein carrying the blood from lungs to left auricle. It has pure blood.
- The blood vessel carrying the blood from the heart towards the body is called artery.
- In artery there is pure blood i.e. oxygen mixed blood. Its exception is pulmonary artery.
- Pulmonary artery carries the blood from right ventricle to lungs. It contains impure blood.
- The artery carrying blood to the muscles of the heart are called coronary arteries. Any type of hindrance in it cause heart attack.

Course of circulation: Mammals have double circulation. It is because blood have to cross two times from heart before circulating throughout body.

- To pump out blood, the heart chamber undergoes alternate contraction called **systole** and relaxation called **diastole.**
- Arteries carry **pure blood** from the heart while veins carry **impure blood** to the heart.
- Human heartbeat is myogenic in nature, i.e., initiated by a patch of modified heart muscles itself without requiring an external stimulation. This patch is called **SA node** (sino-auricular node) or **pacemaker.**
- The normal **rate of heartbeat** of a newborn baby is about 140 per minute.
- When SA-node becomes defective, i.e., it does not generate cardiac impulse, it can be cured by surgical grafting of an artificial pacemaker (an electric device) in the chest of the patient. It stimulates the heart electrically at regular intervals.

EXCRETORY SYSTEM

Kidney

- It is bean-shaped, chocolate brown structure lying in the abdomen, one on each side of the vertebral column just below the diaphragm.
- The left kidney is placed in little higher than the right kidney (but reverse in rabbit).
- These form the urine and controls osmotic pressure within the organism with respect to external environment.
- Nephrons are the functional and structural unit of kidney. They contain Bowman's capsule and Henle's loop.
- The process of filtration of liquids into the cavity of Bowman's capsule is called ultrafiltration.
- The main function of the kidneys is purification of blood plasma, i.e. to excrete the unwanted nitrogenous waste substances through urination.
- In the kidneys average 125 ml per minute blood is filtered.

Ureters

- These bring the urine downwards and open into urinary bladder.

Urinary Bladder

- It temporarily stores the urine.

Urethra

- In females, this tube is small and serves as a passage of urine only.
- In males, it is long and functions as a common passage for urine and spermatic fluids.

Urine

- It is pale yellow coloured fluid due to presence of urochrome pigment.
- It is acidic in nature (pH 6.0) and is slightly heavier than water.
- **Chemical composition of urine**: Water is 95-96%, urea is 2% and some other substances like uric acid, creatinine, etc. are 2-3%.
- Kidney stone is calcium oxalate.
  i. **Skin:** Oil glands and sweat glands found in the skin secrete sebum and sweat.
  ii. **Liver:** Liver cells play the main role in excretion by converting and more amino acids and ammonia of blood into urea.
  iii. **Lungs:** The lungs excrete two types of gaseous substances– carbon dioxide and water vapour.

Hemodialysis: Process of removal of excess urea from the blood of patient using artificial kidney.

CENTRAL NERVOUS SYSTEM

- Nervous system is found only in animals and absent in plants.
- Part of the nervous system which keeps control on the whole body and on nervous system itself is called Central Nervous System. The Central Nervous System of human is made up of two parts–Brain and Spinal Cord.
- Brain is covered by a membrane called meninges. It is situated in a bony box called cranium which protects it from external injury.

Brain

- Brain lies in the cranium of skull.
- The functions of brain parts are as follows:
  i. **Cerebrum** leads to consciousness, storage of memory of information.
  ii. **Thalamus** deals with pain, pressure and temperature.
  iii. **Hypothalamus** deals with water balance in body, behavioural patterns of sex, sleep, stress emotions, etc. It also regulates pituitary hormones and metabolism of fat, carbohydrate and water.
  iv. **Midbrain** deals with visual analysis, etc.
  v. **Cerebellum** controls coordination of accurate movements and balancing.
  vi. Medulla oblongata is long connecting part of brain to spinal cord. It deals with control of heartbeats, blood vessels, breathing, salivary secretion and most of reflex and involuntary (uncontrolled) movements.

Spinal Cord

The posterior region of the medulla oblongata is the spinal cord. Its main functions are:

(a) Coordination and control of reflex actions i.e. it works as the centre of the reflex actions.
(b) It carries the waves coming out of the brain.

SKELETAL SYSTEM

(i) Axial Skeleton (80 Bones)

- It includes skull, vertebral column and bones of chest.
- Vertebral column is responsible for the upright position of the human body.

(ii) Appendicular Skeleton (126 Bones)

- Their functions are to make locomotion possible and to protect the major organs of locomotion, digestion, excretion, and reproduction.

i. **Skull:** There are 29 bones in it.

ii. **Vertebral Column:** The vertebral column of the human is made up of 33 vertebrae.

Functions of the Skeletal System

i. To provide a definite shape to the body.

ii. To provide protection to soft parts of the body.

iii. To provide a base to the muscles for joining.

iv. To help in respiration and nutrition.

v. To form Red Blood Corpuscles.

- The total number of bones in a human's body–206
- The total number of bones during childhood–300
- The largest bone of the body–Femur (bone of thigh).
- The smallest bone of the body–Stapes (bone of ear).

☞ **Note:** The muscles and bones are joined together by tendon. The muscle which joins bone to bone is called ligament.

Classification of Hormones

Amines	Peptide hormones	Steroids/sterols	Lipids
Adrenaline	Acth Or Corticotropin	Cortisol	Prostaglandins
Dopamine	Vasopressin	Aldosterone	Leukotrienes
Noradrenaline	Calcitonin	Testosterone	Prostacyclin
Melatonin	Corticotropin-Releasing Hormone (Crh)	Androstenedione	Thromboxane
Serotonin	Erythropoietin (Epo)	Oestrogen	
Thyroxine	Follicle-Stimulating Hormone (Fsh)	Estradiol	
Triiodothyronine	Gastrin	Progesterone	
	Glucagon	Progestins	
	Gonadotropin-Releasing Hormone (Gnrh)	Calcitriol	
	Growth Hormone-Releasing Hormone (GHRH)	(Sterol)	
	Insulin		
	Leptin		
	Luteinizing Hormone (LH)		
	Oxytocin		
	Parathyroid Hormone (PTH)		
	Prolactin (PRL)		

RESPIRATORY SYSTEM

- Respiration is a catabolic process in which the respired oxygen is used in the oxidation of food resulting in the release of energy.

Human Respiratory System

- Overall passage of air in humans is as follows:

Nostrils–Pharynx–Larynx–Trachea–Bronchi–Bronchioles–Alveoli–Cells–Blood.

External Respiration

- It involves inspiration and expiration of air.
- **Inspiration** is the process of intake of air. During inspiration, muscles of the diaphragm contract and diaphragm flatten. The lower ribs are raised upward and outwards, the chest cavity enlarges, the air pressure in the lungs is decreased, air rushes into the lungs.
- **Expiration** is breathing out of air. During expiration, relaxation of muscles of the ribs and diaphragm takes place. Diaphragm again becomes dome-shaped. Chest cavity is reduced and air is forced outward through nose and trachea.

Internal Respiration (Oxidation of Food)

- It is a complex process in which food is broken down to release energy. It is a biochemical phase takes place inside the cell.
- Transportation of oxygen takes place by haemoglobin of blood, whereas transportation of only 10-20% carbon dioxide takes place by haemoglobin of blood.
- Respiration being a catalytic process also **reduces the weight** of the body.

Glucose is oxidised by oxygen reached into the cell. This process is called cellular respiration.

SENSE ORGANS

Eye

It consists of three parts.

1. Sclerotic Layer

- Cornea
- Conjunctiva

2. Choroid Layer

It is the middle layer and consists of:

i. **Pupil:** It changes size as the amount of light changes.

ii. Ciliary body.

iii. **Iris:** It controls the amount of light that enters the eye by changing the size of the pupil.

iv. Lens is a biconvex transparent circular solid part located just behind the iris.

3. Retina

- Light sensitive tissue that lines the back of the eye.
- The image formed on retina is real and inverted.
- Rods are highly sensitive to dim light and contain a reddish purple pigment called rhodopsin.
- Cones are sensitive to bright light, hence differentiate the colours.
- The **fovea centralis** is the area of sharpest vision.
- The **blind spot:** no image is formed in this region.

Eye Defects

- Nearsightedness (Myopia)
- Farsightedness (Hypermetropia)
- Astigmatism
- Presbyopia
- Conjunctivitis

Ear

- Human ear can list in the sound of 60-80 decibel.
- Defects of ear are: **Otalgia ear-ache** (Pain in ear); **Otitis media** (acute infection of middle ear), **labyrinthine** disease (malfunction of inner ear).

Nose (Olfactory Organ)

Olfactory cells

- Dogs have an acute olfactory sense.

NUTRIENTS

- These are metals, non-metals and their salts other than the four elements– carbon, hydrogen, nitrogen and oxygen and constitute about 4% of total body weight.
- Milk, eggs, meat, fruit, food, vegetables, etc. are the sources of minerals.

Nutrition is one of the basic functions of life in which intake of food, digestion, absorption, assimilation are included.

Carbohydrates

Carbohydrates are organic compounds in which the ratio of Carbon, Hydrogen and Oxygen is 1: 2: 1.

Carbohydrates are classified into three major groups:

(a) **Monosaccharides:** These are the simple sugar made up of single polyhydroxy or ketone unit. Most abundant monosaccharides found in nature are glucose. Triose, tetrose, pentoses, heptoses are the type of monosaccharides.

(b) **Oligosaccharides:** When 2 to 10 monosaccharides join together they form oligosaccharides. Maltose, sucrose, lactose are disaccharides made up of two monosaccharides.

(c) **Polysaccharides:** These are the compounds of sugar which are formed due to joining large number of monosaccharide. Some examples of polysaccharides are starch, glycogen, cellulose, chitin, etc.

Functions of Carbohydrates

1. Carbohydrate works as fuel during the process of respiration, glucose break into CO_2 and H_2O with the release of energy. One gram of glucose gives 4.2 kilo calories energy.
2. Nucleic acids are polymers of nucleosides and nucleotides and contain pentose sugar.
3. Lactose of milk is formed from glucose and galactose.
4. Glucose is used for the formation of fat and amino acid.
5. Carbon skeleton of monosaccharides is used in the formation of fatty acid, chitin, cellulose, etc.

Sources of Carbohydrates

Wheat, rice, maize, sweet potato and other plant and animals are the sources of carbohydrate.

Proteins

- This is a complex organic compound made up of 20 types of amino acids.
- Nitrogen is present in protein in addition to C, H and O.
- Twenty-two types of protein is necessary for human body, out of which 12 are synthesized by body itself and remaining 10 are obtained by food are called essential amino acid.
- These are the compounds of carbon (C), hydrogen (H), oxygen (O), nitrogen (N) and sulphur (S). These form 15% part of human body.
- Their main sources are groundnuts, soyabean, pulses, fish, etc.

Functions of Proteins

1. It takes part in the formation of cells, protoplasm and tissues.
2. These are important for physical growth. Physical growth hampers by their deficiency. Lack of proteins causes Kwashiorkor and Marasmus diseases in children.
3. In case of necessity they provide energy to the body.
4. They control the development of genetic characters.
5. These are helpful in conduction also.

Kwashiorkor: In this disease hands and legs of children get slimmed and the stomach comes out.

Marasmus: In this disease muscles of children are loosened.

Fats

- Fat is an ester of glycerol and fatty acid.
- Normally fat remains as solid at 20°C temperature, but if it is in liquid form at this temperature, this is called oil.
- 9.3 kilocalorie energy is liberated from 1 gram fat.
- These are also the compounds of carbon (C), hydrogen (H) and oxygen (O).
- Fatty acids are of two types. Saturated and Unsaturated. Saturated fatty acids are found in coconut oil and palm oil, while unsaturated fatty acids are found in fish oil and vegetable oil.
- Excess of saturated fats raises the level of blood cholesterol and may cause arteriosclerosis (hardening of arteries). This may lead to heart attack.

Main Functions of Fat

1. It provides energy to the body.
2. It remains under the skin and prevents the loss of heat from the body.
3. It makes the food material tasty.
4. It protects different parts of the body from injury.

- Due to the lack of fat skin gets dried, weight of the body decreases and the development of the body checked.
- Due to the excessiveness of fat the body gets fatty, heart disease takes place and blood pressure increases.

Roughage

- Roughage is another term for dietary fibre, e.g., natural food, *dalia*, etc.
- Helps in retaining water in the body.

Vitamins

It was first invented by FG Hopkins. However, the term vitamin was coined by **C Funk.**

- They provide no calories, they only regulate chemical reactions occurring in the metabolism of the body.
  - i. **Vitamin soluble in water:** Vitamin-B and Vitamin-C.
  - ii. **Vitamin soluble in fat:** Vitamin-A, Vitamin-D, Vitamin-E and Vitamin-K.
- Cobalt is found in Vitamin-B12.
- Synthesis of vitamins cannot be done by the cells and it is fulfilled by the vitamin foods.
- However, synthesis of Vitamin-D and K takes place in our body.
- Synthesis of Vitamin-D takes place by the ultraviolet rays present in the sunlight through cholesterol (ergesterol) of skin.
- Vitamin-K is synthesized in our colon by the bacteria and from there it is absorbed.

Vitamin	Chemical Name	Solubility	Deficiency Disease	Food Sources
Vitamin A	Retinol	Fat	Night blindness	Orange, ripe, yellow fruits, leafy vegetables, carrots, pumpkin, fish, soymilk, milk
Vitamin B_1	Thiamine	Water	Beriberi	Pork, oatmeal, brown rice, vegetables, potatoes, liver, eggs
Vitamin B_2	Riboflavin	Water	Ariboflavinosis, Glossitis	Dairy product, bananas, popcorn, green beans
Vitamin B_3	Niacin, Nicotinomide	Water	Pellagra	Meat, fish, eggs, mushrooms, seeds, nuts
Vitamin B_5	Pantothenic	Water	Parestheria	Meat, broccoli, avocados
Vitamin B_6	Pyridoxine	Water	Anemia	Meat, true nuts, bananas
Vitamin B_7	Priotin	Water	Dematitis, enteritis	Raw egg yolk, liver, peanuts, leafy green vegetables
Vitamin B_8	Folic acid	Water	Megalobastic anemia	Leafy vegetables, pasta, bread, coreal.
Vitamin B_{12}	Cyanocobalamin	Water	Pernicious anemia	Meat, poultry, fish, eggs, milk
Vitamin C	Ascorbic acid	Water	Scurvy	Many fruits and vegetables
Vitamin D	Cholecalciferol	Fat	Rickets	Fish, eggs, liver, mushrooms
Vitamin E	Tocopherols	Fat	Sterility in males and miscarriage in females	Many fruits and vegetables, nuts and seeds
Vitamin K	Phylloquinone	Fat	Bleeding disthesis	Leafy green vegetables, egg yolks

Minerals

These control the metabolism of body.

Water

65-75% weight of the body is water.

Main Functions of Water

1. Water controls the temperature of our body by sweating and vaporizing.
2. It is the important way of excretion of the waste substances from the body.
3. Most of the organic chemical reactions in our body are performed through hydrolysis.

Diseases

Diseases Caused by Protozoa:

- i. **Diarrhoea:** The reason of this disease is the presence of internal protozoa, namely *Entamoeba histolytica* which is spread through houseflies.
- ii. **Filaria:** This disease is caused by *Wuchereia baoncrofti*. This is circulated by the stings of *culex* mosquitoes. This disease is also known as Elephantiasis.

Diseases Caused by Fungus

- i. **Asthma:** This spore of the fungi, namely *Aspergillus fumigate* reaches the lungs of the human and constitutes a net-like formation, thus obstructs the function of lungs. This is an infectious disease.
- ii. **Athlete's foot:** This disease is caused by the fungi namely *Tenia pedes*.
- iii. **Scabies:** This disease is caused by the fungi, namely *Acarus scably*.
- iv. **Baldness:** This is caused by the fungi, namely *Taenia capitis*.
- v. **Ringworm:** This disease spreads through the fungi namely *Trycophyton lerucosum*. This is an infectious disease.

Deficiency Diseases

Deficiency	Diseases	Comments
Vitamin A (retinol)	Xeropthalmia Dermatosis	Lachrimal glands stop producing tears leading to blindness.
(Vitamin B_1) Thiamine	Beri-Beri	Extreme weakness, swelling, pain in legs, loss of appetite, enlarged heart, headache and shortness of breath.
(Vitamin B_2) Riboflavin	Ariboflavinosis	Blurred vision, burning of the eye and tongue, cracking of skin at angle of mouth.
(Vitamin B_3) Niacin (Nicotinamide)	Pellagra,Glossits	Tip and lateral margins of tongue, mouth and gums become red, swollen and develop ulcers
(Vitamin B_5) Pentothenic Acid	Achromotrichia	
Pyridoxine (Vitamin B_6)	Abnormal Protein Metabolism	
(Vitamin B_7) Pantothenic Acid Biotin	Dermatitis, enteritis and anaemia	
(Vitamin B_9) Folic and Folinic Acid	Megaloblast and Birth defects	
(Vitamin B_{12}) Cyanocobalamin	Pernicious or Megaloblastic Anaemia	Reduction of Haemoglobin due to disturbance in the formation of RBC.
Vitamin C (Ascorbic acid)	Scurvy	Pain in joints, loss of weight, gums become spongy and bleed Teeth loose and fragile.
Vitamin D (Cholecalciferol)	Rickets Osteomalacia	Occurs in Children. Softness and deformities of bones Bones susceptible to fracture.
Vitamin E (Tocopherol)		
Vitamin K (Phylloquinone)		
Potassium	Hypokalaemia	Rise in heart beat rate Kidney damage.
Sodium	Hyponatraemia	Low blood pressure.
Proteins	Kwashiorkor	Potbelly due to retention of water by the cells (Oedema).

Diseases caused by Microorganisms

Virus	Bacteria	Protozoas	Fungi	Worms
Small Pox	Sore throat	Malaria	Ringworm	Taeniasis
Chicken Pox	Diphtheria	Amoebic dysentery	Athlete's Foot	Schistosomiasis
Common Cold	Pneumonia	Trypanosomiasis	Madura Foot	Bilharziasis
Influenza/Flu	Tuberculosis	Oriental Sore	Dhobie Itch	Ancylostomiasis
Measles	Plague	Kala Azar		Hookworm
Mumps	Tetanus	Giardiasis		Ascariasis
Encephalitis	Typhoid	Diarrhoea		Enterobiasis
Poliomyelitis	Cholera	Vaginitis		Pinworm disease
Rabies	Bacillary Dysentery			Filariasis
Dengue	Whooping Cough			Elephantiasis
Herpes	Gonorrhoea			
AIDS	Leprosy Botulism			

Hormones

Gland	Hormone	Effect
Pituitary/Hypophysis Anterior Lobe	Growth Hormone or Somatotrophic Hormone (STH)	Growth of long bones, muscles.
	Thyroid Stimulating Hormone (TSH)	
	Adrenocorticotrophic Hormone (ACTH)	Influences the production of corticosteroids by adrenal cortex involved in defending body against physiological stress.
	Follicle-stimulating Hormone (FSH)	Growth and maturation of follicles in the ovary, production of female sex hormone estrogen and maturation of spermatozoa in males..
	Luteinizing Hormone (LH)	Stimulates interstitial cells in the testis to produce testosterone. Causes ovulation. Release of estrogen & formulation of corpus luteum in female.
	Prolactin or Luteotrophic Hormone (LH)	Helps to maintain pregnancy. Stimulate mammary glands to secrete milk.
Middle Lobe	Melanophore-stimulating Hormone (MSH)	Associated with melaonophyte which gives skin its colour.
Posterior Lobe	Vasopressin or Anti-diuretic Hormone	Controls water reabsorption in the kidney tubule.
	Oxytocin	Causes uterine contractions and active expulsion of milk during and after birth.
Hypothalamus	Releasing Hormone (RH) for each anterior pituitary hormone: GH-RH, TSH-RH, ACTH-RH, FSH-RH and likewise	Production of all the anterior pituitary hormones is controlled by messages from the hypothalamus via hypophyseal portal vessels.
Thyroid	Thyroxine/Calcitonin	BMR influences heat production, Calcium level in blood.
Parathyroids	Parathormone	Raises blood calcium level.
Adrenals	Aldosterone	Regulates sodium and potassium levels in the blood to control blood pressure.
	Hydrocortisone	Plays key role in stress response; increases blood glucose levels and mobilises fat stores; reduces inflammation.
	Epinephrine or Adrenalin	Increases blood pressure, heart and metabolic rate, and blood sugar levels; dilates blood vessels. Also released during exercise
	Norepinephrine/Noradrenalin	Increases blood pressure and heart rate; constricts blood vessels.
Thymus	Thymosin	Development of white blood cells.
Pancreas	Insulin Glucagon	Controls blood sugar level. Increase the blood sugar level
Ovaries	Estrogen	Secondary sexual characteristics.
	Progesterone	Prepares Endometrium (inner lining of Uterus) and maintains it during pregnancy.

Exercise

1. **Which programming language is developed by James A Gosling?**
   (a) ASP.Net (b) Java
   (c) PHP (d) C#
2. **Kaleidoscope was invented by ______.**
   (a) John Barber
   (b) Tim Berners-Lee
   (c) Alan Blumlein
   (d) David Brewster
3. **The nitrogenous waste of Human Beings is**
   (a) Ammonia
   (b) Urea
   (c) Ammonium Nitrate
   (d) Uric Acid
4. **Haustoria or sucking roots are found in which of the following?**

(a) Wheat (b) Mango
(c) Chestnut (d) Cuscuta

5. **Equus Asinus is the scientific name of**
(a) Donkey (b) Cow
(c) Deer (d) Kangaroo

6. **______ is an anaesthetic agent.**
(a) Acetylene
(b) Glycol
(c) Diethylether
(d) Ethylene

7. **______ is used for making chemical apparatus like beakers, flasks etc.**
(a) Potash glass
(b) Hard glass
(c) Soda glass
(d) Jena glass

8. **When ice floats on water, its _____ part remains outside the water.**
(a) 0.5 (b) 0.3
(c) 0.1 (d) 1

9. **Instrument for measuring low temperatures is called**
(a) Diagometer
(b) Cryometer
(c) Chromatoptometer
(d) Cymometer

10. **Which drug is used as an Anti-Anxiety drug?**
(a) Warfarin (b) Diazepam
(c) Latanoprost (d) Hydralazine

11. ***Ficus benghalensis* is the scientific name of ______.**
(a) Banyan (b) Pineapple
(c) Babul (d) Tulsi

12. ***Equus burchellii* is the scientific name of ______.**
(a) Horse (b) Zebra
(c) Buffalo (d) Ass

13. **Atomic number of which of the following elements is greater than that of Copper?**
(a) Iron (b) Chromium
(c) Zinc (d) Manganese

14. **Vacuum Tubes were used by _____Generation of Computers.**
(a) First (b) Second
(c) Third (d) Fourth

15. **Which of the following is false with reference to a photo-voltaic cell?**
(a) It is another name for solar cell
(b) It can be used as infra-red detectors
(c) It can store light energy in the form of electrical energy
(d) It converts electric energy into light energy

16. **Methane, an air pollutant is produced _______.**
(a) by action of ultraviolet light on nitrogenous compounds.
(b) as a by-product of manufacturing ammoniacal fertilizers.
(c) by burning of coal in insufficient air.
(d) by digestion of food by animals.

17. **Which drug is used as an Anti-biotic?**
(a) Metformin
(b) Ranitidine
(c) Azithromycin
(d) Ibuprofen

18. ***Tamarindus indica* is the scientific name of ________.**
(a) Neem (b) Pineapple
(c) Tamarind (d) Chiku

19. **In eukaryotic cells synthesis of RNA takes place in the ________.**
(a) mitochondria
(b) centrioles
(c) ribosomes
(d) nucleus

20. **The modern periodic table consists of 18 groups and 7 periods. What is the atomic number of the element placed in the 2nd group and the 4th period?**
(a) 20 (b) 22
(c) 18 (d) 10

21. **Which of the following elements has the lowest melting point?**
(a) Zinc (b) Titanium
(c) Sulphur (d) Fluorine

22. **In Computers, what does ALU stand for?**
(a) Advanced Logic Unit
(b) Accelerated Logic Unit
(c) Arithmetic Logic Unit
(d) Asymmetric Logic Unit

23. **_____ is caused by parasites of the Plasmodium genus.**
(a) Dysentery
(b) Malaria
(c) Chickenpox
(d) Herpes

24. **Who invented Aerosol can?**
(a) Erik Rotheim
(b) Erik Mathew
(c) Erik Tim
(d) Eric Flayer

25. **A transformer can do all of the following except**
(a) step-up a/c voltage
(b) step-up a/c current
(c) step-up a/c power
(d) step-down a/c voltage

26. **What is the unit of the physical quantity "Magnetic field strength"?**
(a) joule per meter
(b) newton per meter
(c) kelvin per meter
(d) ampere per meter

27. ***Acinonyx jubatus* is the scientific name of**
(a) Bear (b) Horse
(c) Cheetah (d) Zebra

28. **Atomic number of which of the following elements is greater than that of Zinc?**
(a) Copper (b) Iron
(c) Chromium (d) Bromine

29. **Commonly used abbreviation SEO in computer science stands for?**
(a) System Engine Optimization
(b) Search Engine Optimization
(c) Structured Engine Optimization
(d) Single Engine Optimization

30. **Who invented Java Script, the programming language?**
(a) Brendan Eich
(b) Willem Einthoven
(c) George Eastman
(d) Emil Erlenmeyer

31. **_______ of a material is defined as the minimum amount of the work necessary to remove a free electron from the surface of the material.**
(a) The electro-repulsive force
(b) The coulomb factor
(c) The power factor
(d) The work function

32. **Human beings' hearing range is**
(a) 50 to 50,000 Hz
(b) 40 to 40,000 Hz
(c) 30 to 30,000 Hz
(d) 20 to 20,000 Hz

33. **Which drug is used as a Thyroid Hormone?**
(a) Metformin
(b) Ketoconazole
(c) Promethazine
(d) Levothyroxine

34. **Which of the following constitute to form a gene?**
(a) Polynucleotides
(b) Hydrocarbons
(c) Lipoproteins
(d) Lipids

35. **Atomic number of which of the following elements is greater than that of Iron?**

(a) Manganese
(b) Cobalt
(c) Calcium
(d) Chromium

36. A series of instructions written by a programmer according to a given set of rules or conventions is called_____.
(a) Syntax (b) a Byte
(c) a Set (d) Macro

37. Who invented LCD Projector?
(a) Gene Dolgoff
(b) Brendan Eich
(c) Douglas Engelbart
(d) Federico Faggin

38. A cannon ball is fired. The motion of this ball is an example of______.
(a) straight line motion
(b) projectile motion
(c) hyperbolic motion
(d) horizontal motion

39. What is the unit of the physical quantity, Magnetic flux?
(a) farad (b) weber
(c) tesla (d) henry

40. Vertebrates belongs to the phylum
(a) Arthropoda (b) Annelida
(c) Cnidaria (d) Chordata

41. What is washing soda?
(a) Aluminium bicarbonate
(b) Sodium bicarbonate
(c) Aluminium sulphate
(d) Sodium carbonate

42. _____is a drug or substance that makes you feel relaxed and makes your body work and react more slowly.
(a) Antidote
(b) Analgesic
(c) Antihistamine
(d) Depressant

43. *Carica papaya* is the scientific name of
(a) Peepal (b) Papaya
(c) Tamarind (d) Drumstick

44. Muscles get tired when there is shortfall of
(a) Lactic acid (b) Na^+ ions
(c) ATP (d) Sulphates

45. The chemical formula of Ammonium nitrate is
(a) $(NHB)_2NO_3$ (b) NH_4NO_3
(c) $NH_4(NOC)_2$ (d) NH_2NO_3

46. Which of the following elements has the lowest melting point?
(a) Xenon (b) Iodine
(c) Barium (d) Magnesium

47. Who invented Induction Coil?
(a) Edwin Howard Armstrong
(b) John Barber
(c) Edwin Beard Budding
(d) Nicholas Callan

48. Find the power of a convex lens if the image formed is at a distance of 16 cm from the lens when the object is placed on the other side of the lens at 2 cm from the optical centre.
(a) –3.75 diopters
(b) –11.25 diopters
(c) 3.75 diopters
(d) 11.25 diopters

49. What is the unit of the physical quantity "Inductance"?
(a) weber (b) farad
(c) henry (d) tesla

50. ______ is a drug that doctors give to people to make them calm or help them sleep.
(a) Barbiturate
(b) Antidepressant
(c) Antihistamine
(d) Beta-Blocker

51. *Artocarpus integra* is the scientific name of ________.
(a) Guava (b) Pineapple
(c) Silver Oak (d) Jackfruit

52. Which organ stores fat soluble vitamins?
(a) Blood (b) Skin
(c) Liver (d) Pancreas

53. Fe has 26 protons in its nucleus. What are the number of electrons in Fe_2^+ (II) ion?
(a) 24 (b) 26
(c) 28 (d) 13

54. Which of the following elements has the lowest melting point?
(a) Titanium (b) Sulphur
(c) Argon (d) Zinc

55. ALU is a part of a computer is ______.
(a) Application (b) ROM
(c) RAM (d) Processor

56. Who invented the 3-D printer?
(a) Nick Holonyak
(b) Elias Howe
(c) Chuck Hull
(d) Christiaan Huygens

57. Alpha particles are ________.
(a) twice the mass of beta particles.
(b) negatively charged.
(c) just like helium nuclei.
(d) lower in ionizing power as compared to gamma rays.

58. Unit of impedance is. _______.
(a) ohm (b) henry
(c) tesla (d) hertz

59. Which disease is caused due to deficiency of Iodine?
(a) Rickets
(b) Scurvy
(c) Goitre
(d) Growth retardation

60. *Grevillea robusta* is the scientific name of
(a) Peepal (b) Teak
(c) Silver Oak (d) Jack fruit

61. The Modern Periodic Table consists of 18 groups and 7 periods. What is the atomic number of the element placed in the 3rd group and the 4th period?
(a) 23 (b) 21
(c) 19 (d) 11

62. Which of the following elements has the lowest melting point?
(a) Oxygen (b) Gold
(c) Silver (d) Manganese

63. Who is known as father of computer?
(a) Charles Babbage
(b) Tim Berners Lee
(c) Douglas Carl Engelbart
(d) Sabeer Bhatia

64. Who discovered X-Ray?
(a) Wilhelm Rontgen
(b) William Lee
(c) X Rollswick
(d) I Thompson

65. Find the power of a convex lens if the image formed is at a distance of 25 cm from the lens when the object is placed on the other side of the lens at 12 cm from the optical centre?
(a) – 4.33 diopters
(b) 12.33 diopters
(c) – 12.33 diopters
(d) 4.33 diopters

66. What is the unit of the physical quantity 'Entropy'?
(a) watt per kelvin
(b) newton per kelvin
(c) pascal per kelvin
(d) joule per kelvin

67. Kidney stones are composed of
(a) Calcium Oxalate
(b) Sodium Chloride
(c) Magnesium Nitrate
(d) Calcium Bicarbonate

68. Which of the following is not true about Angiosperms?
(a) Dominant phase is gametophytes
(b) Vascular bundles are present
(c) Spores are heterospores
(d) Seeds are covered

69. All of the following are excretory (waste) products of animals, except
(a) Uric Acid
(b) Ammonia
(c) Carbohydrates
(d) Urea

70. RNA is a polymeric molecule. What does RNA stand for?
(a) Rado Nuclear Acid
(b) Ribo Nucleic Acid
(c) Rhino Nuclear Acid
(d) Resto Nucleus Acid

71. The common name of dichlorodifl- uoromethane is
(a) galena (b) freon
(c) gypsum (d) borax

72. _______performs tasks such as inserting, updating, or deleting data occurrences.
(a) Data definition language
(b) Data manipulation language
(c) Query language
(d) OQL

73. Who invented the computer mouse?
(a) Gene Dolgoff
(b) Brendan Eich
(c) Douglas Engelbart
(d) Federico Faggin

74. _______ states that internal energy is a function of state and the increase in internal energy is equal to the sum of the heat supplied to system and work done by the system.
(a) First law of thermodynamics
(b) Hooke's Law
(c) The coulomb's law
(d) Faraday's Law

75. What is the direction of torque?
(a) Perpendicular to the direction of applied force
(b) Same as the direction of applied force
(c) Opposite to the direction of applied force
(d) Parallel to the radius

76. Which organ does detoxification and produces chemicals needed for digestion?
(a) Salivary glands
(b) Pancreas
(c) Thyroid gland
(d) Liver

77. $NaHCO_3$ is chemical formula for
(a) Borax (b) Vinegar
(c) Lime (d) Baking soda

78. Which of the following elements has the lowest melting point?
(a) Chromium (b) Hydrogen
(c) Zinc (d) Silver

79. C Programming language was developed by
(a) Charles Babbage
(b) Larry Wall
(c) James Gosling
(d) Dennis Ritchie

80. Instrument for measuring blueness of the sky or ocean is called
(a) Bathymeter (b) Ceraunograph
(c) Cyanometer (d) Barometer

81. Farad is unit of _______.
(a) Capacitance
(b) Reactance
(c) Electric charge
(d) Electric conductance

82. Which drug is used to cure Incontinence?
(a) Oxybutynin
(b) Ranitidine
(c) Azithromycin
(d) Levothyroxine

83. In which part of the cell are proteins made?
(a) reticulum
(b) Golgi apparatus
(c) ribosomes
(d) lysosome

84. Polio is a disease caused by which of the following?
(a) Bacteria (b) Mosquito
(c) Virus (d) Cockroach

85. Chemical formula of Ammonia is
(a) PH_3 (b) NO_2
(c) AlN (d) NH_3

86. Which of the following elements has the lowest melting point?
(a) Oxygen (b) Platinum
(c) Sodium (d) Tin

87. Find the power of a convex lens if the image formed is at a distance of 20 cm from the lens when the object is placed on the other side of the lens at 25 cm from the optical centre.
(a) 1 diopters (b) –9 diopters
(c) 9 diopters (d) –1 diopters

88. What is the unit of the physical quantity "Capacitance"?
(a) weber (b) farad
(c) tesla (d) ohm

89. The outer white part of the eye that protects the inner structures is
(a) Iris (b) Sclera
(c) Retina (d) Cornea

90. Proteins are made up of _______.
(a) Amino acids
(b) Fatty acids
(c) Glucose
(d) Nucleotides

91. The Modern Periodic Table consists of 18 groups and 7 periods. What is the atomic number of the element placed in the 4th group and the 4th period?
(a) 24 (b) 20
(c) 22 (d) 12

92. A Gigabyte equals all of the following, except _______.
(a) 1000 megabytes
(b) trillion bytes
(c) Million kilobytes
(d) 1 thousandth of a terabyte

93. Who discovered Catalysis?
(a) Messcureni (b) Berzelius
(c) Hooke (d) Garner

94. Find the power of a convex lens if the image formed is at a distance of 20 cm from the lens when the object is placed on the other side of the lens at 60 cm from the optical centre.
(a) 3.33 diopters
(b) 6.67 diopters
(c) – 6.67 diopters
(d) – 3.33 diopters

95. What is the unit of the physical quantity "Heat capacity"?
(a) watt per kelvin
(b) joule per kelvin
(c) newton per kelvin
(d) pascal per kelvin

96. *Moringa oleifera* is the scientific name of ________.
(a) Banyan (b) Gulmohar
(c) Amla (d) Drumstick

97. ________ is a drug that makes your heart work more slowly, used for treating high blood pressure.
(a) Contraceptive
(b) Beta-Blocker
(c) Depressant
(d) Enema

98. *Ocimum tenuiflorum* is the scientific name of ________.
(a) Neem (b) Mango
(c) Babul (d) Tulsi

99. Which gland secretes bile, a digestive fluid?
(a) pancreas (b) liver
(c) thyroid (d) testes

100. The chemical formula of ammonium chloride is ________.
(a) $(NHD)_2Cl$ (b) NH_4Cl_3
(c) NH_4Cl_2 (d) NH_4Cl

101. Which of the following elements has the lowest melting point?
(a) Iron (b) Nitrogen
(c) Iodine (d) Lead

102. In Internet, what is the full form of TCP ?
(a) Transfer Control Program
(b) Transfer Control Protocol
(c) Transmission Control Program
(d) Transmission Control Protocol

103. Pyrolusite is an ore/mineral of ________.
(a) Mercury
(b) Manganese
(c) Molybdenum
(d) Lead

104. Who invented Internet Protocol?
(a) Vint Cerf
(b) David Chaum
(c) Georges Claude
(d) Josephine Cochrane

105. Find the power of a convex lens if the image formed is at a distance of 10 cm from the lens when the object is placed on the other side of the lens at 40 cm from the optical centre.
(a) 12.5 diopters
(b) 7.5 diopters
(c) – 12.5 diopters
(d) – 7.5 diopters

106. Filament of electric bulb is made of ________.
(a) Magnesium (b) Lead
(c) Tin (d) Tungsten

107. The amount of blood filtered together by both the kidneys in a 70 kg adult male human in a minute is
(a) 1100 ml (b) 100 ml
(c) 1500 ml (d) 500 ml

108. Which feature of a plant helps to distinguish a monocot from a dicot?
(a) pollination (b) venation
(c) vernation (d) aestivation

109. The Mutation Theory was proposed by ________.
(a) Charles Lyell
(b) William Smith
(c) Hugo De Vries
(d) Harrison Schmitt

110. Which of the following elements has the lowest melting point?
(a) Helium (b) Potassium
(c) Tungsten (d) Sulphur

111. Atomic number of which of the following elements is greater than that of Phosphorus?
(a) Aluminium (b) Silicon
(c) Chlorine (d) Magnesium

112. The designers of the Internet Protocol defined an IP address as a ________ bit number.
(a) 8 (b) 16
(c) 32 (d) 64

113. Which type of pathogen causes the water-borne disease Hepatitis-A?
(a) Parasitic (b) Viral
(c) Protozoan (d) Bacterial

114. ________ is a natural electrical phenomenon characterized by the appearance of streamers of reddish or greenish light in the sky, especially near the northern or southern magnetic pole.
(a) Acaulis (b) Alatus
(c) Albopictus (d) Aurora

115. Who invented Laser?
(a) William Friese-Greene
(b) Arthur Fry
(c) Gordon Gould
(d) Otto von Guericke

116. What is the SI unit of Torque?
(a) newton/meter
(b) newton meter
(c) newton second
(d) newton/meter squared

117. What is the unit of the physical quantity, Illuminance?
(a) siemens (b) tesla
(c) lux (d) weber

118. *Arboreal ateles* is the scientific name of ________.
(a) Squirrel (b) Sparrow
(c) Lizard (d) Spider monkey

119. The chemical formula of Ammonia is ________.
(a) NH (b) NH_4
(c) NH_2 (d) NH_3

120. Who discovered Fullerene (an allotrope of carbon)?
(a) K Scheele
(b) Richard Smalley
(c) Faraday
(d) Heisenberg

121. ________ perform Internet Protocol blocking to protect networks from unauthorized access.
(a) Firewalls (b) Proxy Servers
(c) Routers (d) VoIP

122. Which type of pathogen causes the waterborne disease Salmonellosis?
(a) Algal (b) Parasitic
(c) Bacterial (d) Viral

123. Which of the following is not a Halon gas?
(a) methane
(b) Carbon tetrachloride
(c) iodomethane
(d) bromomethane

124. If a body moves with a uniform speed in a circular motion, then ________.
(a) its acceleration is increasing
(b) its acceleration is zero
(c) its velocity is changing
(d) its velocity is uniform

125. ________ is the fourth state of matter.
(a) Plasma (b) Steam
(c) Gas (d) Matteroid

126. Blood leaving the liver and moving towards the heart has a higher concentration of ________.
(a) Lipids
(b) Urea
(c) Bile Pigments
(d) Carbon dioxide

127. Bulb is a modification of which part of a plant?
(a) The root (b) The stem
(c) The radicle (d) The fruit

128. Which of the following carries blood away from the heart to different body parts?
(a) Arteries (b) Nerves
(c) Capillaries (d) Veins

129. Chemical formula of water is ________.
(a) O_2H (b) OH
(c) HO (d) H_2O

130. Atomic number of which of the following elements is greater than that of Aluminium?
(a) Phosphorus (b) Neon
(c) Magnesium (d) Sodium

131. Which of these is not a web browser?
(a) Chrome (b) Firefox
(c) Safari (d) Linux

132. Who invented dishwasher?
(a) Vint Cerf
(b) David Chaum
(c) Georges Claude
(d) Josephine Cochrane

133. ________states that the induced e.m.f. is directly proportional to the rate of change of magnetic flux linkage or rate of cutting of magnetic flux linkage.
(a) Lenz's Law (b) Hooke's Law
(c) Ohm's Law (d) Faraday's Law

134. If the vector sum of torques acting on a system is zero, then the object is in ________.
(a) static equilibrium
(b) translatory equilibrium
(c) linear equilibrium
(d) rotational equilibrium

135. BCG vaccine is given to protect from which of the following?
(a) Jaundice
(b) Anaemia
(c) Tuberculosis
(d) Polio

136. Parallel venation is found in ________.
(a) plants which are monocots
(b) plants which have a dicot stem
(c) plants with leaves similar to Tulsi
(d) plants with tap roots

137. The hardest part of the body is ________.
(a) Bones (b) Tooth Enamel
(c) Skull (d) Spinal Cord

138. The Chemical formula of Ammonium sulphate is
(a) NH_4SO_4 (b) $(NHD)_2SO_3$
(c) NH_4SO_3 (d) $(NHD)_2SO_4$

139. The common name of lead (II) sulphide is
(a) borax (b) epsom salt
(c) galena (d) brimstone

140. SMTP in computer science stands for?
(a) Simple Markup Transfer Protocol
(b) Systems Mail Transfer Protocol
(c) Simple Mail Transfer Protocol
(d) Systems Memory Transfer Protocol

141. Which type of pathogen causes the waterborne disease, E. coli Infection?
(a) Protozoan (b) Parasitic
(c) Bacterial (d) Viral

142. ________is a measure of the actual amount of water vapour in a particular sample of air: measured as a partial pressure.
(a) Specific Humidity
(b) Absolute Humidity
(c) Relative Humidity
(d) Dew Point

143. Who Invented Lawnmower?
(a) Edwin Howard Armstrong
(b) John Barber
(c) Edwin Beard Budding
(d) Nicholas Callan

144. ________is defined as the force acting per unit current per unit length on a wire placed at right angles to the magnetic field.
(a) Magnetic susceptibility
(b) Magnetic flux density
(c) Magnetic flux
(d) Magnetic pulse

145. If an object moves in a purely rotatory motion, then each constituent particle of the body moves in a circle, the centre of which is located on a line is called ________.
(a) the axis of rotation
(b) the line of rotation
(c) the spinning rod
(d) the fixed line

146. Which of the following is a primary function of haemoglobin?
(a) Utilization of energy
(b) Prevention of anaemia
(c) Destruction of bacteria
(d) To transport oxygen

147. Vascular bundles are absent in________.
(a) Bryophyta
(b) Pteridophyta
(c) Gymnosperms
(d) Angiosperms

148. *Sauria lacertidae* is the scientific name of________.
(a) Crocodile (b) Hippopotamus
(c) Lizard (d) Housefly

149. In chemistry, soap is a salt of a ______.
(a) Fatty acid
(b) Glycol
(c) Phosphorus
(d) Ammonium Carbonate

150. A ________ is a pair of forces, equal in magnitude, oppositely directed, and displaced by perpendicular distance or moment.
(a) bond (b) couple
(c) pair (d) duo

151. Which of these is not an Operating System?
(a) Android (b) iOS
(c) HTML (d) Symbian

152. Which type of pathogen causes the water-borne disease SARS (Severe Acute Respiratory Syndrome)?
(a) Viral (b) Parasitic
(c) Protozoan (d) Bacterial

153. Excessive richness of nutrients in a lake or other body of water is called _____.
(a) Biomagnification
(b) Global Warming
(c) Salination
(d) Eutrophication

154. Who Invented Aspirin?
(a) Ruth Handler
(b) John Harington
(c) Rowland Hill
(d) Felix Hoffmann

155. A larger force on a rotating body results in larger _____.
(a) mass
(b) torque

(c) axis of rotation
(d) centre of mass

156. What is the unit of the physical quantity, Magnetic flux density?
(a) siemens (b) weber
(c) henry (d) tesla

157. The fat digesting enzyme Lipase is secreted by which of the following?
(a) Kidneys
(b) Pancreas
(c) Large Intestine
(d) Liver

158. The arrangement of leaves on an axis or stem is called
(a) phyllotaxy (b) vernation
(c) venation (d) phytotaxy

159. The study of Cells is also known as
(a) Cytology (b) Physiology
(c) Nucleology (d) Cellology

160. The Chemical formula of Urea is
(a) $(NH_4)_2CO_2$ (b) $(NH_2)CO$
(c) $(NH_4)_2CO$ (d) $(NH_2)_2CO$

161. Atomic number of which of the following elements is greater than that of Magnesium?
(a) Neon (b) Fluorine
(c) Sodium (d) Aluminium

162. TCP in computer science stands for?
(a) Transmission Control Protocol
(b) Total Control Protocol
(c) Technology Control Protocol
(d) Transfer Control Protocol

163. Who invented water turbine?
(a) Enrico Fermi
(b) Adolf Gaston Eugen Fick
(c) Sandford Fleming
(d) Benoit Fourneyron

164. _______ of a wave is the rate of transfer of energy per unit area perpendicular to the direction of travel of the wave.
(a) Interference (b) Rectification
(c) Intensity (d) Diffraction

165. Motion of a train is an example of ______.
(a) Rotatory motion
(b) Spin motion
(c) Projectile motion
(d) Translatory motion

166. Deficiency of which vitamin causes night blindness?
(a) Vitamin K (b) Vitamin C
(c) Vitamin B_1 (d) Vitamin A

167. The flower with the world's largest bloom is _____.
(a) Pando
(b) Posidonia
(c) *Rafflesia arnoldii*
(d) *Helianthus annuus*

168. The scientist who proposed the cell theory was
(a) Schleiden and Schwann
(b) Lamarck
(c) Treviranus
(d) Whittaker and Stanley

169. ______ decreases the rate of setting of cement.
(a) Alumina
(b) Silica
(c) Gypsum
(d) Magnesium oxide

170. Alkenes were earlier known as ______.
(a) Paraffins (b) Titoffins
(c) Olefins (d) Meloffins

171. A language used to control the tasks of the computer itself, such as starting other programs, is _____.
(a) Command Language
(b) Machine Language
(c) Markup Language
(d) Style Sheet Language

Answers

1. (b)	**2.** (d)	**3.** (b)	**4.** (d)	**5.** (a)	**6.** (c)	**7.** (b)	**8.** (c)	**9.** (d)	**10.** (b)
11. (a)	**12.** (b)	**13.** (c)	**14.** (a)	**15.** (d)	**16.** (d)	**17.** (c)	**18.** (c)	**19.** (d)	**20.** (a)
21. (d)	**22.** (c)	**23.** (b)	**24.** (a)	**25.** (c)	**26.** (d)	**27.** (c)	**28.** (d)	**29.** (b)	**30.** (a)
31. (d)	**32.** (d)	**33.** (d)	**34.** (a)	**35.** (b)	**36.** (a)	**37.** (a)	**38.** (b)	**39.** (b)	**40.** (d)
41. (d)	**42.** (d)	**43.** (b)	**44.** (c)	**45.** (b)	**46.** (a)	**47.** (d)	**48.** (d)	**49.** (c)	**50.** (a)
51. (d)	**52.** (c)	**53.** (a)	**54.** (c)	**55.** (d)	**56.** (c)	**57.** (c)	**58.** (a)	**59.** (c)	**60.** (c)
61. (b)	**62.** (a)	**63.** (a)	**64.** (a)	**65.** (b)	**66.** (d)	**67.** (a)	**68.** (a)	**69.** (c)	**70.** (b)
71. (b)	**72.** (b)	**73.** (c)	**74.** (a)	**75.** (a)	**76.** (d)	**77.** (d)	**78.** (b)	**79.** (d)	**80.** (c)
81. (a)	**82.** (a)	**83.** (c)	**84.** (c)	**85.** (d)	**86.** (a)	**87.** (c)	**88.** (b)	**89.** (b)	**90.** (a)
91. (c).	**92.** (b)	**93.** (b)	**94.** (b)	**95.** (b)	**96.** (d)	**97.** (b)	**98.** (d)	**99.** (b)	**100.** (d)
101. (b)	**102.** (d)	**103.** (b)	**104.** (a)	**105.** (a)	**106.** (d)	**107.** (a)	**108.** (b)	**109.** (c)	**110.** (a)
111. (c)	**112.** (c)	**113.** (b)	**114.** (d)	**115.** (c)	**116.** (b)	**117.** (c)	**118.** (d)	**119.** (d)	**120.** (b)
121. (a)	**122.** (c)	**123.** (a)	**124.** (c)	**125.** (a)	**126.** (c)	**127.** (b)	**128.** (a)	**129.** (d)	**130.** (a)
131. (d)	**132.** (d)	**133.** (d)	**134.** (d)	**135.** (c)	**136.** (a)	**137.** (b)	**138.** (d)	**139.** (c)	**140.** (c)
141. (c)	**142.** (b)	**143.** (c)	**144.** (b)	**145.** (a)	**146.** (d)	**147.** (a)	**148.** (c)	**149.** (a)	**150.** (b)
151. (c)	**152.** (a)	**153.** (d)	**154.** (d)	**155.** (b)	**156.** (d)	**157.** (b)	**158.** (a)	**159.** (a)	**160.** (d)
161. (d)	**162.** (a)	**163.** (d)	**164.** (c)	**165.** (d)	**166.** (d)	**167.** (c)	**168.** (a)	**169.** (c)	**170.** (c)
171. (a)									

PRACTICE SETS

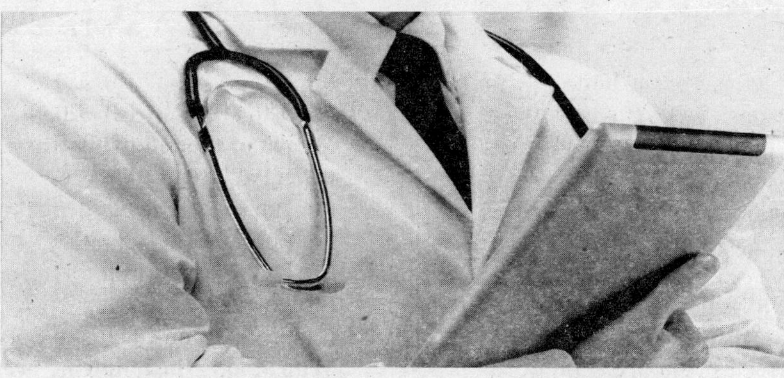

PRACTICE SET-1

1. Who built the Buddhist monuments at Sanchi?
(a) Mughal dynasty
(b) Maurya dynasty
(c) Gupta dynasty
(d) Chola dynasty

2. Gulzar won Oscars for the movie 'Slumdog Millionaire' in the category of
(a) Best sound mixing
(b) Best original score
(c) Best original song
(d) Best foreign language film

3. Which of the following is a primary function of haemoglobin?
(a) Utilisation of energy
(b) Prevention of anaemia
(c) Destruction of bacteria
(d) To transport oxygen

4. Vascular bundles are absent in
(a) Bryophyta (b) Pteridophyta
(c) Gymnosperms (d) Angiosperms

5. Sauria lacertidae is the scientific name of
(a) crocodile
(b) hippopotamus
(c) lizard
(d) house fly

6. In Chemistry, soap is a salt of
(a) fatty acid
(b) glycol
(c) phosphorus
(d) ammonium carbonate

7. A .... is a pair of forces, equal in magnitude, oppositely directed, and displaced by perpendicular distance or moment.
(a) bond (b) couple
(c) pair (d) duo

8. Which of these is not an Operating System?
(a) Android (b) iOS
(c) HTML (d) Symbian

9. Chapchar Kut is a festival of which State?
(a) Manipur (b) Nagaland
(c) Mizoram (d) Meghalaya

10. Who built the Taj Mahal?
(a) Humayun (b) Shah Jahan
(c) Babar (d) Jahangir

11. In which stage of the business cycle the inventory stock will be the highest?
(a) Boom (b) Depression
(c) Recession (d) Recovery

12. Which type of pathogen causes the water-borne disease SARS (Severe Acute Respiratory Syndrome)?
(a) Viras
(b) Parasitic
(c) Protozoan
(d) Bacterial

13. Excessive richness of nutrients in a lake or other body of water is called
(a) Biomagnification
(b) Global Warming
(c) Salination
(d) Eutrophication

14. Which of the following is a Direct tax ?
(a) Excise duty
(b) Customs duty
(c) Service tax
(d) Wealth tax

15. The boundary line between India and Pakistan is called
(a) McMahon line (b) Maginot line
(c) Radcliffe line (d) Sir Creek

16. Which city is located on the banks of the river Mahanadi?
(a) Bengaluru (b) Cuttack
(c) Badrinath (d) Kota

17. When was the battle of Haldighati fought?
(a) 1776 (b) 1676
(c) 1576 (d) 1476

18. In 1498, which Portuguese explorer discovered a new sea route from Europe to India?
(a) Vasco da Gama
(b) Christopher Columbus
(c) Sir Francis Drake
(d) John Cabot

19. Who invented Aspirin?
(a) Ruth Handler
(b) John Harington
(c) Rowland Hill
(d) Felix Hoffmann

20. A larger force on a rotating body results in larger
(a) mass
(b) torque
(c) axis of rotation
(d) centre of mass

21. What is the unit of the physical quantity, magnetic flux density?
(a) Siemens (b) Weber
(c) Henry (d) Tesla

22. Article-24 of the Indian Constitution 'Prohibition of employment of children in factories, etc. deals with
(a) fundamental rights of the Indian Citizen
(b) Union government
(c) State government
(d) Directive principles of State policy

23. Article-134A of the Indian Constitution 'Certificate for appeal to the Supreme Court' deals with
(a) State government
(b) Union government
(c) Fundamental rights of the Indian citizen
(d) Directive principles of State policy

24. Highest number of test hundreds is scored by
(a) Jacques Kallis
(b) Sachin Tendulkar
(c) Ricky Ponting
(d) Brian Lara

25. Who is the author of 'Can Love Happen Twice'?
(a) Keshav Aneel
(b) Ravinder Singh
(c) Sudeep Nagarkar
(d) Aravind Adiga

26. Schedule VII of the Indian Constitution contains
(a) Presidential election
(b) Acts beyond judicial review
(c) States and union territories
(d) Division of Powers into 3 lists

27. Which Article of the Indian Constitution mentions about financial emergency?
(a) 360 (b) 350
(c) 340 (d) 330

28. Which of the following was not an aspect of later Vedic Age?
(a) Importance of kingship in political life
(b) Discovery of iron
(c) Polygamy
(d) Simple, non-ritualistic worship

29. Who among the following presided over the fourth Buddhist Council?
(a) Ashoka (b) Kanishka
(c) Ashvaghosha (d) Vasumitra

30. Which of the following was not built by Firoz Shah Tughlaq?
(a) Firozabad (b) Fatehabad
(c) Tughlaqabad (d) Jaunpur

Answers with Explanations

1. (b) The 'Great Stupa' at Sanchi is the oldest structure and was originally commissioned by the emperor Ashoka the Great in the 3rd century BCE. Ashoka belonged to the Mauryan Empire and most of the Buddhist monuments were build during this period only.

2. (c) Gulzar won Oscars in the category of Best Original Song for the song 'Jai Ho' in movie named Slumdog Millionaire.

3. (d) The major function of haemoglobin is to transport oxygen from the lungs to the body's tissues and then transport carbon dioxide out of the tissue back to the lungs.

4. (a) Bryophyta, traditional name for any nonvascular seedless plant. In contrast to vascular plants, the bryophyte sporophyte usually lacks a complex vascular system and produces only one spore-containing organ (sporangium) rather than many.

5. (c)

Scientific Name	Animal
Sauria lacertidae	Lizard
Crocodylus niloticus	Crocodile
Hippopotamus amphibious	Hippopotamus
Musca domestica	House fly

6. (a) Soap is produced by a saponification or basic hydrolysis reaction of fat or oil. Currently, sodium carbonate or sodium hydroxide is used to neutralise the fatty acid and convert it to the salt.

7. (b)

8. (c) Operating System is the low-level software that supports a computer's basic functions, such as scheduling tasks and controlling peripherals. Hypertext Markup Language (HTML), a standardised system for tagging text files to achieve font, colour, graphic, and hyperlink effects on World Wide Web pages. All others are operating systems.

9. (c) The Chapchar Kut is a festival of Mizoram, India. It is celebrated during March after completion of their most arduous task of Jhum operation i.e., jungle-clearing (clearing of the remnants of burning). It is a spring festival celebrated with great fervor and gaiety.

10. (b)

11. (b) In Economics, a depression is a sustained, long-term downturn in economic activity in one or more economies. The value of money depreciates in this phase which leads to increase in Inventory stock.

12. (a) SARS is caused by a member of the coronavirus family of viruses (the same family that can cause the common cold). It is believed that the 2003 epidemic started when the virus spread from small mammals in China. When someone with SARS coughs or sneezes, infected droplets spray into the air.

13. (d) Eutrophication refers to the excessive richness of nutrients in a lake or other body of water, frequently due to run-off from the land, which causes a dense growth of plant life.

Biomagnification, also known as bioamplification or biological magnification, is the increasing concentration of a substance, such as a toxic chemical, in the tissues of organisms at successively higher levels in a food chain. Global Warming is the increase of Earth's average surface temperature due to effect of greenhouse gases, such as carbon dioxide emissions from burning fossil fuels or from deforestation, which trap heat that would otherwise escape from Earth.

14. (d) A tax, such as income tax, which is levied on the income or profits of the person who pays it, rather than on goods or services is called as direct tax. Key examples of direct taxes are Income tax, Wealth tax, Corporation tax.

15. (c) The Radcliffe Line was published on August 17, 1947 as a boundary demarcation line between India and Pakistan upon the Partition of India. It was named after its architect, Sir Cyril Radcliffe, who as chairman of the Border Commissions. McMahon line is between India and China. Sir Creek is a 96 km tidal estuary on the border of India and Pakistan. The Creek, which opens up into the Arabian Sea, divides the Gujarat State of India from the Sindh province of Pakistan. The Maginot Line named after the French Minister of War Andre Maginot, was a line of concrete fortifications, obstacles, and weapon installations built by France in the 1930s to deter invasion by Germany. Constructed on the Fench side of its borders with Switzerland, Germany, and Luxembourg.

16. (b)

City	River
Bengaluru	Vrishabhavathi
Cuttack	Mahanadi
Badrinath	Alaknanda
Kota	Chambal

17. (c) The Battle of Haldighati was fought in Haldighati, Rajasthan on June 18 or 21, 1576 for around four hours between Rana of Mewar, Maharana Pratap and Mughal Emperor Akbar's forces led by Man Singh I.

18. (a) The discovery of the sea route to India is the description sometimes used in Europe and among the Portuguese for the first recorded trip made directly from Europe to India via the Atlantic Ocean. It was undertaken under the command of Portuguese explorer Vasco da Gama during the reign of King Manuel I in 1497-1499.

19. (d) Felix Hoffmann, a German chemist, produced a stable form of acetylsalicylic acid, more commonly known as aspirin, in 1897. Aspiring is used to reduce fever and relieve mild to moderate pain from conditions such as muscle aches, toothaches, common cold, and headaches. Aspirin is known as a salicylate and a nonsteroidal anti-inflammatory durg (NSAID).

20. (b)

21. (d)

Physical Quantity	Unit
Electyrical Conductance	Siemens
Magnetic flux	Weber
Inductance	Henry
Magnetic flux Density	Tesla

22. (a) Article-24 mandates that no child below age of 14 years shall be employed to work any factory or mine or engaged in any other hazardous employment. Article-(12-35) deals with the fundamental rights of the citizen of India.

23. (b)

24. (b) Sachin Tendulkar has scored 100 centuries (100 or more runs) in Test matches and One Day International (ODI) matches, organised by the International Cricket Council. His total of 51 centuries in Test matches and 49 in ODIs is a world record for highest number of centuries by a batsman.

25. (b)

26. (d) Seventh Schedule (Article 246) provides for the division of powers between the Union of India and the states. It deals with the union (central government), state, and concurrent lists of responsibilities. The lists have been called Union List, State List and Concurrent List.

27. (a) Article 360 of the Indian Constitution deals with financial emergency. If the President is satisfied that there is an economic situation in which the financial stability or credit of India is threatened, he or she can declare financial emergency. Such an emergency must be approved by the Parliament within two months.

28. (d) In the early Vedic period, religious practice was in the form of nature worship. However, the focus shifted to rituals and sacrifices during the later Vedic period. Religious practices were refined and worship of Gods in the form of idols gained importance. With rituals and hymns taking centerstage, the evolution of Hindu religion took place.

29. (d) The fourth Buddhist Council is said to have been convened by the Kushan emperor Kanishka in Kashmir in 78 CE. For this council, Kanishka gathered 500 monks headed by Vasumitra. The main fruit of this Council was the vast commentary known as the Maha-Vibhasha.

30. (c) Tughlaqabad was a heavy fortified city built by Ghiyasuddin Tughlaq, the founder of Tughlaq dynasty, in 1321. The city was built to keep away the Mongol marauders.

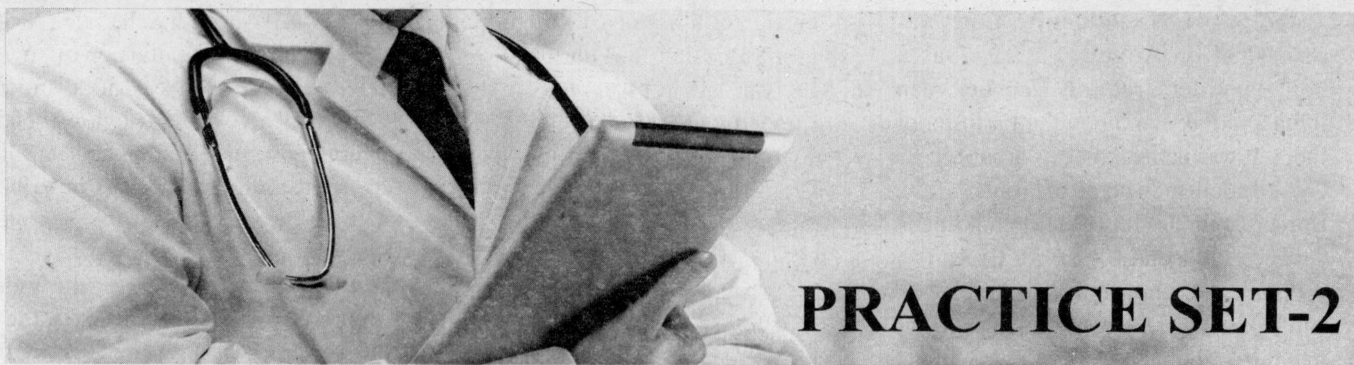

PRACTICE SET-2

1. Chemical formula of washing soda is
(a) $Na_2SO_4.10H_2O$ (b) $NaHCO_3$
(c) $Na_2CO_3.10H_2O$ (d) $Ca(OH)_2$

2. Hydrochloric acid is also known as
(a) Galic acid (b) Picric acid
(c) Muriatic acid (d) Chloric acid

3. Khangchendzonga National Park is located at
(a) Uttar Pradesh
(b) West Bengal
(c) Sikkim
(d) Jammu and Kashmir

4. Biosphere Reserve of India Nanda Devi is located in the state of
(a) Uttarakhand
(b) Sikkim
(c) Meghalaya
(d) Himachal Pradesh

5. In a desert region, soil erosion can be checked by
(a) Contour ploughing
(b) Using farm manure
(c) Tree plantation/Afforestaion
(d) Crop rotation

6. The first oil refinery in India was set up at
(a) Barauni
(b) Vishakhapatnam
(c) Digboi
(d) Mumbai

7. The chemical name of baking soda is
(a) Sodium carbonate
(b) Sodium bicarbonate
(c) Sodium chloride
(d) Sodium nitrate

8. The name of the train "Shatabdi Express" refers to the centenary of
(a) Mahatma Gandhi
(b) Indian National Congress
(c) India's War of Independence
(d) Jawaharlal Nehru

9. Which one of the following is not a rabi crop ?
(a) Mustard (b) Rice
(c) Wheat (d) Gram

10. The driest part of India is
(a) Western Rajasthan
(b) Jammu and Kashmir
(c) Gujarat
(d) Madhya Pradesh

11. "Mumbai High" is associated with
(a) Steel (b) Petroleum
(c) Mausoleum (d) Jute

12. Which one of the following goods has only exchange value ?
(a) Diamond (b) Television
(c) Computer (d) Rice

13. The power to decide an Election Petition for the State is vested in the
(a) Parliament
(b) Supreme Court
(c) High Courts
(d) Election Commission

14. How many items are there in the Union List?
(a) 52 (b) 66
(c) 97 (d) 99

15. What is the maximum gap permissible between two sessions of Parliament?
(a) One month
(b) Three months
(c) Six months
(d) Twelve months

16. When were the Fundamental Duties incorporated in the Constitution?
(a) 1975 (b) 1976
(c) 1977 (d) 1979

17. The number of Nationalised Banks in India is
(a) 14 (b) 21
(c) 20 (d) 22

18. Rift Valley is formed
(a) between two anticlines
(b) between two faults
(c) erosion of synclinal basin
(d) due to volcanic eruption

19. Lake formed by Aswan Dam in Africa is
(a) Chad (b) Victoria
(c) Nasser (d) Tanganyika

20. How many judges are there in Supreme Court ?
(a) 25 (b) 26
(c) 30 (d) 31

21. During the reign of Bindusara there was unrest at
(a) Ujjayani
(b) Pushkalavati
(c) Taxila
(d) Rajagriha

22. Widening of a river valley takes place due to
(a) Corrosion
(b) Lateral erosion
(c) Corrasion
(d) Hydraulic action

23. Water of coconut is
(a) liquid nucellus
(b) liquid mesocarp
(c) liquid endocarp
(d) degenerated liquid endosperm

24. Bulbils takes part in
(a) Sexual reproduction
(b) Vegetative reproduction
(c) Food storage
(d) Respiration

25. Fish is a first class protein as it contains
(a) essential amino-acids
(b) non-essential amino acids
(c) all essential fatty acids
(d) no amino acid

26. Who among the following granted permission to the English to establish their factory in India?
(a) Akbar (b) Jehangir
(c) Shah Jahan (d) Aurangzeb

27. Which of the following regions is called the 'granary of the world'?
(a) Temperate grasslands
(b) British-type vegetation
(c) Laurentian-type vegetation
(d) Tropical grasslands

28. Which of the following rivers of India flows in the rift valley?
(a) Kaveri (b) Tapti
(c) Son (d) Ken

29. Yeasts bring about fermentation by the action of a complex enzyme known as
(a) invertase (b) catalase
(c) peroxidase (d) zymase

30. Name the gland which has both exocrine and endocrine functions.
(a) Liver (b) Thymus
(c) Pituitary (d) Pancreas

Answers with Explanations

1. (c) Washing Soda is essentially Sodium Carbonate, a sodium salt of carbonic acid (soluble in water). The molecular formula of washing soda is $Na_2CO_3.10H_2O$. It is used as an agent to soften hard water. It reacts with the calcium and magnesium bonds present in the water, enabling the detergent to work.

2. (c) Hydrochloric acid was historically called acidum salis, muriatic acid, and spirits of salt because it was produced from rock salt and green vitriol and later from the chemically similar substances common salt and sulfuric acid. Hydrochloric acid is found naturally in gastric acid.

3. (c) Khangchendzonga National Park is locate in Sikkim. The park gets its name from the mountain Khangchendzonga which is 8,586 metres tall, the third-highest peak in the world. The park is known for animals like musk deer, snow leopard and Himalayan Thar.

4. (a) The Nanda Devi National Park (Biosphere Reserve) is situated around the peak of Nanda Devi, in Uttarakhand. It was established in 1982. Along with the adjoining Valley of Flowers National Park, it was inscribed a World Heritage Site by UNESCO in 1988.

5. (c) Afforestation holds the key for preventing soil erosion in desert regions and further desertification. Trees or even small plants bind soil to their roots, thereby checking their loosening. Some other measures include: introduction of improved dry farming practices and animal husbandry and plantations for fuel and fodder.

6. (c) Digboi in Tinsukia district of Assam has the distinction of having the oldest oil refinery of India and Asia as well. It was here that the first commercially viable well in India, well No.1, was successfully drilled in September 1889 and first modern refinery in India was built and commissioned in December 1901 by Assam Oil Company Ltd.

7. (b) Sodium bicarbonate ($NaHCO_3$) is also known as baking soda. It is a chemical leavening agent which is added to baked goods before cooking to produce carbon dioxide and cause them to 'rise'.

8. (d) The word "Shatabdi" means centenary in Sanskrit, Hindi and several Indian languages. The first Shatabdi train was started in 1988 to commemorate the centenary of Pandit Jawahar Lal Nehru's Birthday (the First Prime Minister of India) by Madhav Rao Scindia, minister for railways. It operated from New Delhi to Jhansi, later extended to Bhopal.

9. (b) Rabi refers to agricultural crops sown in winter and harvested in the spring. Examples of Rabi Crops: Wheat, Gram, Pea, Mustard, Linseed, Barley. Rice is a Kharif crop, cultivated and harvested during the rainy (monsoon) season in the South Asia.

10. (a) Western Rajasthan is the driest region in India. Jaisalmer in western Rajasthan is the driest place which receives the lowest rainfall (less than 10 cm). It is due to its distance from the monsoon winds of the Bay of Bengal and location in the sub-tropical high pressure belt.

11. (b) Bombay High, also known as Mumbai High, is an offshore oilfield 162 kilometres off the coast of Mumbai about 75 m of water. The oil operations are run by India's Oil and Natural Gas Corporation (ONGC).

12. (a) Adam Smith argued that although water has no value in exchange it has considerable value in use, while a diamond has no value in use but considerable value in exchange. It is known as Paradox of value. This distinction was associated with a belief that only physical things could have a value and that labour was the source of all value.

13. (c) Section 80-A of the Representation of the People Act, 1951 provides that the High Court shall be the authority for presentment of election petitions under Article 329(b) of the Constitution. This was incorporated by an amendment in the year 1966 (Act 47 of 1966).

14. (c) The Union List or List-I is a list of 100 items (though last item is numbered 97) given in Part XI of the Constitution of India on which Parliament has exclusive power to legislate. Out of the 100 items on the list, one is no longer in force.

15. (c) The Constitution empowers the President to summon each House at such intervals that there should not be more than 6-month's gap between the two sessions. Hence the Parliament must meet at least twice a year. In India, the parliament conducts three sessions each year.

16. (b) The Forty Second Constitution Amendment Act, 1976 has incorporated ten Fundamental Duties in Article 51(a) of the Constitution of India. This was done in accordance with the recommendation of the Sardar Swaran Singh Committee. India adopted Fundamental Duties from the Constitution of erstwhile USSR.

17. (c) On July 19, 1969, 14 commercial banks were nationalized, which got presidential approval on August 9, 1969. In 1980, in order to provide government more power and command over credit delivery, six more commercial banks in India were nationalized.

18. (b) A rift valley is a linear shaped lowland between several highlands or mountain ranges created by the action of a geologic rift or fault. It is formed by the subsidence of a segment of the Earth's crust between dip-slip, or normal, faults.

19. (c) Lake Nasser was created by the construction of the Aswan High Dam in Southern Egypt across the waters of the Nile between 1958 and 1971. The largest man-made lake in the world, Lake Nasser has a major role in Egypt's fishing industry.

20. (d) As originally enacted, the Constitution of India provided for a Supreme Court with a Chief Justice and 7 judges. As the work of the Court has increased, the present sanctioned strength has swelled to 31.

21. (c) During the reign of Bindusara, Chandragupta Maurya's son and successor, there was unrest at Taxila in the north-western province of Sindh. He sent Asoka (his son) to quell the uprising. Taxila was a highly volatile place because of the Indo-Greek presence and mismanagement of Governor Susima.

22. (b) Lateral or sideways erosion widens the river valley; while, Vertical or downward erosion deepens the river valley. Due to continued lateral erosion, the river valley increasingly becomes broader and shallower. The valley slopes are also eroded by weathering and mass wasting and by the development of tributary valleys.

23. (d) Coconut water, the clear liquid inside young green coconuts (fruits of the coconut palm), is liquid endosperm. In early development, it serves as a suspension for the endosperm of the coconut during their nuclear phase of development. It contains sugars, vitamins, minerals, proteins, free amino acids and growth promoting factors.

24. (b) Bulbil is a small bulblike organ of vegetative reproduction growing in leaf axils or on flower stalks of plants such as the onion and tiger lily. It is a reproductive organ that takes part in vegetative reproduction. The bulbils drop from the parent plant on to the ground, give out adventitious roots and develop into new plants.

25. (a) Animal proteins derived from meat and fish are called first class proteins. A first class protein is one which contains all 8 essential amino acids (which cannot be made by the body). They are also called complete proteins. Plant proteins are called second class proteins.

26. (b) Mughal Emperor Jahangir gave permission for an English factory at Surat in 1619. He granted them permission to trade in his territories at Surat (in Gujarat) on the west coast and Hughli (in West Bengal) in the east. This permission was given during the visit of Captain William Hawkins to the imperial court.

27. (a) Temperate grasslands are ideal for extensive wheat cultivation and produce the huge surplus of wheat per capita amongst the world's wheat growing nations. The Prairie is known as the 'Granary of the World' due to surplus wheat production.

28. (b) Narmada and Tapi rivers flow in the geological faults (rifts) created between two ancient mountain ranges, 'Vindhya' and 'Satpura'. It is also noteworthy that while most of the rivers originate from east and flow towards south or south-west, Narmada and Tapi Rivers flow from east to west because of the faulted zones and drain into Arabian Sea.

29. (d) Zymase is an enzyme complex that catalyses the fermentation of sugar into ethanol and carbon dioxide. It occurs naturally in yeasts. Zymase activity varies among yeast strains.

30. (d) The pancreas has two main functions: an exocrine function that helps in digestion and an endocrine function that regulates blood sugar. The pancreas contains exocrine glands that produce enzymes important to digestion. The endocrine component of the pancreas consists of islet cells that create and release important hormones directly into the bloodstream. Two of the main pancreatic hormones are insulin, which acts to lower blood sugar, and glucagon, which acts to raise blood sugar.

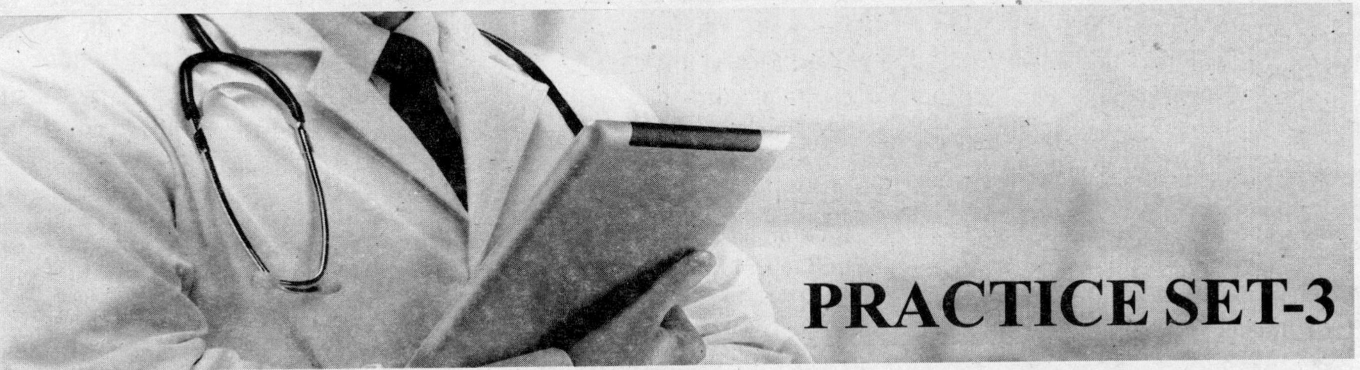

PRACTICE SET-3

1. The most suitable soil for the production of cotton is :
(a) Black lava soil
(b) Alluvial soil
(c) Loamy soil
(d) Well drained soil

2. In which region of electromagnetic spectrum does the Lyman series of hydrogen atom lie ?
(a) Visible (b) Infrared
(c) Ultraviolet (d) X-ray

3. Perfectly inelastic demand is equal to :
(a) One
(b) Infinite
(c) Zero
(d) Greater than one

4. The largest producer of Lignite in India is :
(a) Kerala (b) Tamil Nadu
(c) Rajasthan (d) Gujarat

5. Impeachment Proceedings against the President for violation of the Constitution can be initiated in :
(a) Either House of Parliament
(b) The Lok Sabha
(c) The Rajya Sabha
(d) The Supreme Court

6. Who is the first woman IPS officer in India ?
(a) Sarojini Naidu
(b) Kiran Bedi
(c) Indira Gandhi
(d) Bachendri Pal

7. In operationg system, Round Robin Scheduling means :
(a) A kind of scheduling
(b) Repetition policy
(c) A memory allocation policy
(d) A process allocation policy

8. Soldering of two metals is possible because of the property of:
(a) Viscosity
(b) Osmosis
(c) Cohesion
(d) Surface tension

9. December 1 is celebrated as :
(a) Indian Navy Day
(b) UNICEF Day
(c) World AIDS Day
(d) Children's Day

10. Which one of the following tribes practices pastoral nomadism?
(a) Boro (b) Masai
(c) Pygmies (d) Eskim

11. The 73rd Constitutional amendment act is related to:
(a) Foreign Exchange
(b) Finance Commission
(c) Panchayat Raj
(d) RBI

12. Which state of India has made rain water harvesting compulsory for all houses?
(a) Haryana (b) Maharashtra
(c) Tamil Nadu (d) Punjab

13. FORTRAN is called :
(a) Formula Translator
(b) Format Translator
(c) File Translator
(d) Floppy Translator

14. The area reserved for the welfare of wildlife is called:
(a) Sanctuary
(b) Forest
(c) National Park
(d) Botanical garden

15. The famous activist Medha Patkar is associated with which movement ?
(a) Beti Bachao, Beti Padhao Yojana
(b) Narmada Bachao Andolan
(c) Preserve the wetlands
(d) Save the Tiger

16. Whose army did Alexander, the Greek ruler confront on the banks of the river Jhelum?
(a) Chandragupta Maurya
(b) Ambi
(c) Dhanananda
(d) Porus

17. Which of the following is the right expansion of ILO?
(a) International Law and Order
(b) Inter-State Lawful Ordinance
(c) Indian Legal Orientation
(d) International Labour Organization

18. Ryder Cup is a famous tournament of:
(a) Lawn Tennis (b) Badminton
(c) Cricket (d) Golf

19. The National Green Tribunal deals with cases relating to :
(a) Issues relating to protection and conservation of historical monuments.
(b) Civil cases
(c) Criminal offences
(d) Environmental protection and conservation of forests.

20. Maximum oxygen comes from:
(a) Deserts
(b) Green forests
(c) Grass lands
(d) Phytoplanktons

21. Kanha National Park is located in :
(a) Bihar
(b) Madhya Pradesh
(c) Andhra Pradesh
(d) TmilNadu

22. Sex-ratio is calculated as :
(a) No. of children per 1,000 people in a Country.
(b) No. of males per 1,000 females in a Country.
(c) No. of females per 1,000 males in a Country.
(d) No. of people per 1,000 children in a Country.

23. Project tiger programme was launched in :
(a) 1975 (b) 1973
(c) 1994 (d) 1971

24. Who built "Old Fort" ?
(a) Akbar (b) Shershah
(c) Aurangzeb (d) Babar

25. Where did Chandragupta Maurya spent his last days?
(a) Pataliputra
(b) Thaneshwar
(c) Kanchi
(d) Shravanabelagola

26. How many states are there in the Indian Union?
(a) 27 (b) 28
(c) 30 (d) 29

27. The Battle of Plassey was fought between
(a) Sirajud-Daulah and Robert Clive.
(b) None of the options
(c) Mir Kasim and Robert Clive.
(d) Mir Jafar and Robert Clive.

28. In which year was the first World Environment Day observed?
(a) 1972 (b) 1980
(c) 1973 (d) 1974

29. Which of the following properties of sound is affected by change in air temperature?
(a) Frequency (b) Intensity
(c) Amplitude (d) Wavelength

30. Soilless agriculture refers to
(a) Hydroponics
(b) Hygroponics
(c) Sericulture
(d) Inter-cropping

Answers with Explanations

1. (a) Black soil is most suitable for the cultivation of cotton. The deep and medium black lava soil of the Deccan and Malwa plateaus is considered ideal, though it can be grown on alluvial and red soil as well. The black cotton soil is also known as regur.

2. (c) In Physics and Chemistry, the Lyman series is a hydrogen spectral series of transitions and resulting ultraviolet emission lines of the hydrogen atom as an electron goes from $n > 2$ to $n = 1$ (where n is the principal quantum number), the lowest energy level of the electron. The first line in the spectrum of the Lyman series was discovered in 1906 by Harvard physicist Theodore Lyman, while studying the ultraviolet spectrum of electrically excited hydrogen gas. The rest of the lines of the spectrum (all in the ultraviolet) were discovered by Lyman from 1906-1914.

3. (c) Price Elasticity of Demand is a measure of the relationship between a change in the quantity demanded of particular goods and a change in its price. It measures the responsiveness of demand to changes in price for particular goods. If the price elasticity of demand is equal to 0, demand is perfectly inelastic (i.e., demand does not change when price changes).

4. (b) State-wise distributions of Indian Lignite shows that major parts of the resource are located in Tamil Nadu followed by Rajasthan, Gujarat, Pondicherry, J & K, Kerala, and West Bengal. About 75 percent of lignite production in India comes from Neyveli in Tamil Nadu.

5. (a) According to Article 61 of Indian Constitution, when a President is to be impeached for violation of the Constitution, the charge shall be preferred by either House of Parliament. It adds that no such charge shall be preferred unless:

- the proposal to prefer such charge is contained in a resolution which has been moved after at least fourteen days notice in writing signed by not less than one-fourth of the total number of members of the House has been given of their intention to move the resolution, and
- such resolution has been passed by a majority of not less than two-thirds of the total membership of the House.

6. (b) Kiran Bedi became the first woman IPS Officer in India in 1972. Bedi's first posting was to the Chanakyapuri subdivision of Delhi in 1975. The same year, she became the first woman to lead the all-male contingent of the Delhi Police at the Republic Day Parade in 1975.

7. (a) Round robin is the scheduling algorithm used by the CPU during execution of the process. Round robin is designed specifically for time sharing systems. It is similar to first come first serve scheduling algorithm but the preemption is the added functionality to switch between the processes.

8. (c) Soldering is the process of joining two metals by the use of a solder alloy, and it is one of the oldest known joining techniques. It is possible because of the property of cohesion, the interaction between adjacent parts of the same body and as acting throughout the interior of substance. Soldering leads to alloy formation at the layer between two metals.

9. (c) World AIDS Day is held on the 1st December each year. World AIDS Day was first conceived in August 1987 by James W. Bunn and Thomas Netter; the day has been observed since 1988. It is one of the eight official global public health campaigns marked by the World Health Organization (WHO).

10. (c) Pygmies are nomadic hunter-gatherers who live in the equatorial rainforests of central Africa as well as parts of southeast Asia. They are nomadic, and obtain their food through a mix of foraging, hunting, fishing, and trading with inhabitants of neighbouring villages. Their cultural identity is very closely tied to the rainforest, as are their spiritual and religious views.

11. (c) The Constitution (Seventy third Amendment) Act, 1992 is related to Panchayati Raj in India. It added Part IX of the Constitution of India, related to Panchayats, and the Eleventh Schedule to the Constitution which deals with matters on which the Panchayats may be devolved with powers and responsibility by the State Legislatures by law.

12. (c) Rainwater harvesting has been made compulsory for every building in Tamil Nadu to avoid groundwater depletion. Since its implementation, Chennai saw a 50 percent rise in water level in five years and the water quality significantly improved. Rainwater harvesting is the accumulation and deposition of rainwater for reuse on-site, rather than allowing it to run off.

13. (a) Fortran is a general-purpose, imperative programming language that is especially suited to numeric computation and scientific computing. Its name is a contraction of Formula Translation. It aims to provide a way to tell computers to calculate complicated mathematical expressions, with more ease than assembly language.

14. (c) A National Park is an area which is strictly reserved for the welfare of wildlife and where activities such as forestry, grazing or cultivation are not allowed. Private ownership, rights and habitat, manipulation are not permitted in a national park. There are 103 national parks in India covering an area of 40,500 km^2, which is 1.23% of the geographical area of the country.

15. (b) Medha Patkar is an Indian social activist and social reformer turned politician who founded the Narmada Bachao Andolan (NBA) in 1989. It is a social movement consisting of adivasis, farmers, environmentalists, and human rights activists against a number of large dams being built across the Narmada river.

16. (d) The Battle of the Hydaspes was fought by Alexander the Great in 326 BC against King Porus of the Paurava kingdom on the banks of the river Hydaspes (Jhelum) in the Punjab near Bhera. The battle resulted in a complete Macedonian victory and the annexation of the Punjab.

17. (d) Myopia, also known as near-sightedness and shortsightedness, is a condition of the eye where the light that comes in does not directly focus on the retina but in front of it, causing the image that one sees when looking at a distant object to be out of focus, but in focus when looking at a close object.

18. (d) ILO stands for International Labour Organization. It is a United Nations agency dealing with labour issues, particularly international labour standards, social protection, and work opportunities for all. Formed in 1919, it is headquartered in Geneva, Switzerland.

19. (d) The Ryder Cup is a biennial men's golf competition between teams from Europe and the United States. It is contested every two years with the venue alternating between courses in the United States and Europe. The Ryder Cup is named after the English businessman Samuel Ryder who donated the trophy.

20. (d) Most of Earth's oxygen comes from tiny ocean plants - called phytoplankton - that live near the water's surface and drift with the currents. Like all plants, they photosynthesize- that is, they use sunlight and carbon dioxide to make food. Scientists believe that phytoplankton contribute between 50 to 85 percent of the oxygen in Earth's atmosphere.

21. (b) Kanha National Park is the largest national park of Madhya Pradesh. Also known as Kanha Tiger Reserve, it is one of the tiger reserves of India. It was created on 1 June 1955. Kanha provided inspiration to Rudyard Kipling for his famous novel "Jungle Book."

22. (b) Project Tiger is a tiger conservation programme launched in 1973 by the Government of India. The aim of the project was to control as well as supplement the dwindling population of the Royal Bengal tigers in the country. Project Tiger is administered by the National Tiger Conservation Authority.

23. (b) Old Fort is one of the oldest forts in Delhi. Its current form was built by the Afghan king Sher Shah Suri, on a site which was perhaps that of Indraprastha, the legendary capital of the Pandavas. Though Sher Shah began its construction, the monument was completed by his son Islam Shah.

24. (d) During his last days, Chandragupta gave away his throne to his son, Bindusara, and spent his life as an ascetic. He accepted Jainism and spent his last days at Sravanabelagola in Karnataka along with Bhadrabahu. He gave up his life by the strict Jain ritual of sallakhena.

25. (a) Ammonia gas that dissolves in water forms a solution of ammonium hydroxide (NH_4OH). This solution (including the gas) is a strong base and will make the solution alkaline.

$$H_2O + NH_3 \Leftrightarrow OH^- + NH_4^+$$

26. (d) India is a federal union of states comprising twenty-nine states and seven union territories. Telangana split from Andhra Pradesh to become the newest – 29th – State of India on 2nd June] 2014 with Hyderabad as the shared capital.

27. (a) The Battle of Plassey was fought between Nawab Sirajud-Daulah, the last independent Nawab of Bengal, and the British East India Company under Robert Clive on 3rd June, 1757. It resulted in a decisive victory of the British East India Company over the Nawab and his French allies and the establishment of the Company Rule in Bengal.

28. (c) The World Environment Day (WED) was established by the United Nations General Assembly (UNGA) on the day the United Nations Conference on the Human Environment began in Stockholm. Sweden, on 5th June, 1972. The first World Environment Day was hosted in 1973. WED has been celebrated every year on 5th June since then.

29. (d) The wavelength of sound changes with temperature This is because the speed of sound changes with the temperature. Since the speed of sound is different at different temperatures, this means the wavelength of sound at a given frequency is a variable depending on the speed of sound. For example, the wavelength of a 100-cycle tone in air at 68°F would be 11.27 feet while the same tone in fresh water at 68°F would have a wavelength of 48.05 feet.

30. (a) Hydroponics is a subset hydroculture and is a method of growing plants using mineral nutrient solutions in water, without soil. Terrestrial plants may be grown with their roots in the minernutrient solution only, or in an inert medium, such as perlite or gravel. Hydroponics a subset of soilless culture.

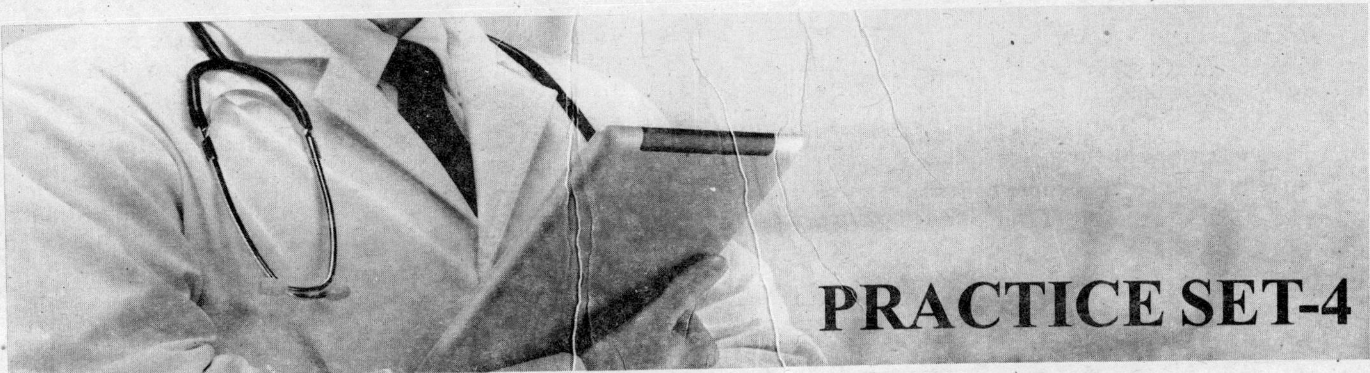

1. **Who is the author of the book "The 3 Mistakes of My Life"?**
   (a) Ruskin Bond
   (b) Chetan Bhagat
   (c) Amrita Pritam
   (d) Jhumpa Lahiri
2. **Who invented the mobile phone?**
   (a) Tim-Berners-Lee
   (b) Raymond Samuel Tomlinson
   (c) Chuck Hull
   (d) Martin Cooper
3. **Who was the creator of the famous Rock Garden of Chandigarh?**
   (a) Khushwant Singh
   (b) Charles Corbusier
   (c) Edward Baker
   (d) Nek Chand
4. **Kathakali dance form is associated with which State?**
   (a) Tamil Nadu
   (b) Andhra Pradesh
   (c) Manipur
   (d) Kerala
5. **According to 2011 Census, the State having maximum population is**
   (a) Maharashtra
   (b) Tamil Nadu
   (c) Kerala
   (d) Uttar Pradesh
6. **Which decade is called as the "Era of Decolonisation"?**
   (a) 1950's (b) 1980's
   (c) 1990's (d) 1970's
7. **Who is the only second Vice-President of India to get a second consecutive term after S. Radhakrishnan?**
   (a) K.R. Narayanan
   (b) B.S. Shekhawat
   (c) Mohammad Hamid Ansari
   (d) Dr. Shankar Dayal Sharma
8. **An ordinance issued by the Governor has to be passed by the Assembly within**
   (a) 8 weeks (b) 10 weeks
   (c) 12 weeks (d) 6 weeks
9. **Who has authored the book "The Kingdom of God is Within You"?**
   (a) Leo Tolstoy
   (b) Henry David
   (c) Mahatma Gandhi
   (d) John Ruskin
10. **Which of the following was the founder of the house of Peshawar?**
    (a) Ramachandra Pant
    (b) Balaji Vishwanath
    (c) Balaji Baji Rao
    (d) Parsuram Triamsuk
11. **Who was the founder of the Indian National Army?**
    (a) Nehru
    (b) Subhash Chandra Bose
    (c) Bal Gangadhar Tilak
    (d) Gandhiji
12. **Which Indian rular fought the Kalinga War?**
    (a) Samudragupta
    (b) Chandragupta
    (c) Shivaji
    (d) Ashoka
13. **Cuba is the largest producer of**
    (a) Barley (b) Sugar
    (c) Wheat (d) Rice
14. **The basic unit of biosystematics is**
    (a) Phenotype (b) Ecotype
    (c) Florotype (d) Genotype
15. **Which endocrine gland is found in chest cavity?**
    (a) Pineal gland
    (b) Thymus gland
    (c) Adrenal gland
    (d) Thyroid gland
16. **An organism that transmits disease from one individual to another is called**
    (a) Hybrid (b) Fragment
    (c) Vector (d) Clone
17. **A semi enclosed coastal body of water which has a free connection with the open sea is called**
    (a) Estuary (b) Fjord
    (c) Cove (d) Ria coast
18. **Which part of the cinchona yields a drug?**
    (a) Pericarp (b) Bark
    (c) Endosperm (d) Leaf
19. **S.I. unit of Magnetic flux is**
    (a) weber (b) weber/m
    (c) weber/m^4 (d) weber-m^2
20. **Which of the following colour of light deviates least through the prism?**
    (a) yellow (b) green
    (c) violet (d) red
21. **An example of hormone is**
    (a) Cytosine (b) Renin
    (c) Oxytocin (d) Peprin
22. **Name the two research stations maintained by India in Antarctica**

(a) Gangotri and Himadri
(b) Sagar Nidhi amd Yamunotri
(c) None of these
(d) Maitri and Bharti

23. The 'EL Nino' phenomena which sparks climatic extreme around the globe, originates in the
(a) Sea of China
(b) Pacific Ocean
(c) Indian Ocean
(d) Atlantic Ocean

24. The term GIGO is related to
(a) Flexibility (b) Versatility
(c) Automatic (d) Accuracy

25. 'Chipko movement' associated with
(a) Saving the tigers
(b) Saving the wetland
(c) None of these
(d) Trees

26. The idea of parliamentary form of government is adapted from
(a) US (b) UK
(c) Ireland (d) USSR

27. How many Nobel Prize awards are awarded each year?
(a) 10 (b) 6
(c) 5 (d) 8

28. Phycology is the study of
(a) Bacteria (b) Algae
(c) Fungi (d) Lichens

29. Who invented the safety razor?
(a) Gillette (b) Steve Cher
(c) Steve Jobs (d) Lar Strauss

30. Barter transactions mean
(a) Goods are exchanged with gold.
(b) Coins are exchanged for goods.
(c) Money acts as a medium of exchange.
(d) Goods are exchanged with goods.

Answers with Explanations

1. (b) 'The 3 Mistakes of My Life' is the third novel written by Chetan Bhagat. The book was published in May 2008. The novel follows the story of three friends and is based in the city of Ahmedabad, Gujarat. The movie version of the novel is Kai Po Che!

2. (d) Martin Cooper, an American engineer, conceived the first handheld mobile phone while at Motorola in 1973. He led the team that developed it and brought it to market in 1983. He is considered the "father of the cell phone" and is also cited as the first person in history to make a handheld cellular phone call in public.

3. (d) The Rock Garden of Chandigarh is a sculpture garden that was created by Nek Chand, a government official who started it secretly in his spare time in 1957. It is also known as Nek Chand's Rock Garden. Today, it is spread over an area of 40 acres. It is completely built of industrial and home waste items.

4. (d) Kathakali originated in the present day state of Kerala during the 17th century. It is a stylized classical Indian dance-drama noted for the attractive make-up of characters, elaborate costumes, detailed gestures and well-defined body movements presented in tune with the anchor playback music and complementary percussion.

5. (d) With total population of 199,281,477, Uttar Pradesh is the most heavily populated state of India as per the 2011 Census. It constitutes 16.49% of India's population. Maharashtra and Bihar come next with respective contributions of 9.28% and 8.58% to the national population.

6. (d) Most historians describe late 1950s as the era of decolonization. It was in this decade that large-scale decolonization in Africa first began. In 1951 Libya became the first African country to gain independence in the decade, and in 1954 the Algerian War began. In 1956, Sudan, Morocco, and Tunisia become independent, and Ghana became the first subsaharan African nation to gain independence in 1957.

7. (c) Mohammad Hamid Ansari is the only second vice-president of India to get a second consecutive term after S. Radhakrishnan. He was elected as Vice President of India on 10 August 2007 and took office on 11 August 2007. He was re-elected on 7 August 2012.

8. (d) As per Article 213 of Indian Constitution, an Ordinance promulgated by the Governor of a state has to be laid before the Legislative Assembly or where there is a Legislative Council in the State, before both the Houses. It ceases to operate at the expiration of six weeks from the reassembly of the Legislature, or if before the expiration of that period a resolution disapproving it is passed by the Legislative Assembly and agreed to by the Legislative Council.

9. (a) The Kingdom of God is Within You is a non-fiction book written by Leo Tolstoy. A philosophical treatise, the book was first published in Germany in 1894 after being banned in his home country of Russia. Gandhi cited the book as one of the most important modern influences in his life.

10. (b) Balaji Vishwanath was the founder of the house of the Peshwas in 1714. He was the first of a series of hereditary Peshwas hailing from the Marathi Chitpavan Brahmin family who gained effective control of the Maratha Empire during the 18th century. He is also called the second founder of the Maratha Empire.

11. (b) The Indian National Army was first formed in 1942 under Mohan Singh, by Indian prisoners of war of the British- Indian Army captured by Japan in the Malayan campaign and at Singapore. However, it soon fell into decline. It was revived under the leadership of Subhas Chandra Bose after his arrival in Southeast Asia in 1943.

12. (d) The Kalinga War was fought between the Mauryan Emperor Ashoka and Raja Anantha Padmanabhan of Kalinga in 262 B.C. It was the only major war Ashoka fought after his accession to throne. However, it is one of the major and bloodiest battles in world history. The bloodshed of this war is said to have prompted Ashoka to adopt Buddhism.

13. (b) Historically, Cuba was the largest producer of sugarcane and one of the leading exporters in the 20th century. It was once known as 'sugar bowl of the world.' However, its place has now been taken by Brazil. At present, Brazil, India and China are the three leading sugar producing countries of the world. Best Choice: (b) Sugar

14. (b) Ecotype is the basic unit of Biosystematics. It is adapted to a particule environment but capable of producing fully fertile hybrids with other ecotypes. The term Ecotype was proposed by Turesson. According to him Ecotype is "an ecological unit to cover the product arising as a result of genotypical response of an ecospecies to a particular habitat."

15. (b) The endocrine glands are widely distributed throughout the body. The pituitary gland, pineal gland and hypothalamus are located in the skull. The thyroid and parathyroid glands are in the neck, and the thymus gland is in the thoracic (chest) cavity. The thymus gland is only active until puberty. It helps the body protect itself against autoimmunity.

16. (c) An organism that transmits a disease agent from an infected to a non-infected animal or plant is known as vector. The major classes of vectors are:

- Non-living vectors (food, water, soil, other materials)
- Arthropod vectors (fleas, ticks, mosquitoes)
- Vertebrate vectors (rats, mice, cats, dogs, birds)

17. (a) An estuary is a semi-enclosed coastal body of water which has a free connection with the open sea and within which seawater is measurably diluted with freshwater derived from land drainage. Estuaries form a transition zone between river environments and maritime environments. They are subject both to marine and riverine influences.

18. (b) The bark of cinchona tree yields quinine, a white crystalline alkaloid having antipyretic (fever-reducing), antimalarial, analgesic (painkilling), and anti-inflammatory properties. Quinine was the first effective Western treatment for malaria caused by Plasmodium falciparum.

19. (a) The SI unit of magnetic flux is the Weber (Wb) (in derived units: volt-seconds). It is the magnetic flux that linking a circuit of one turn, would produce in it an electromotive force of 1 volt if it were reduced to zero at a uniform rate in 1 second. It is named after the German physicist Wilhelm Eduard Weber. The CGS unit of magnetic flux is Maxwell.

20. (d) In refracting media like glass prism, water, etc., lights of different colours travel with different speeds. The speed of violet colour is the least, while the speed of red colour is the largest in prism. As a result, the refractive index of glass is largest for violet colour and least for red colour. So the violet colour is deviated the most, while red colour is deviated least on passing through the prism.

21. (c) Oxytocin is an hormone that is normally produced in the hypothalamus and stored in the posterior pituitary gland. It plays a role in social bonding, sexual reproduction in both sexes, and during and after childbirth. It is released due to stretching of the cervix and uterus during labour and with stimulation of the nipples from breastfeeding.

22. (d) India has three research stations in Antarctica: Dakshina Gangotri, Maitri and Bharati. India's first committed research facility, Dakshin Gangotri, was set up in 1983. It is currently being used as a supply base. Maitri and Bharati were set up in 1989 and 2012 respectively.

23. (b) El Nino (Little Boy, or Christ Child in Spanish) refers to the large-scale oceanatmosphere climate interaction linked to a periodic warming in sea surface temperatures across the central and east-central Equatorial Pacific. It was originally recognized by fishermen off the coast of South America in the 1600s, with the appearance of unusually warm water in the Pacific Ocean.

24. (d) Garbage in, garbage out (GIGO), in the context of information technology, is a slang expression that means regardless of how accurate a program's logic is, the results will be incorrect if the input is invalid. A program gives inaccurate results due to inaccurate data provided because a computer will always attempt to process data given to it. So GIGO is related to accuracy of output which in turn is dependent on the accuracy of inputs.

25. (d) The Chipko movement refers to an organized resistance to the destruction of forests that arose in India during the 1970s. The name of the movement comes from the word 'embrace', as the villagers hugged the trees, and prevented the contractors from felling them. In 1987, the Chipko Movement was awarded the Right Livelihood Award.

26. (b) The Constitution of India provides for a parliamentary form of government, both at the Centre and in the states that has been borrowed from the United Kingdom. The parliamentary government is also known as cabinet government or responsible government or Westminster model of government and is prevalent in Japan, Canada, among others.

27. (b) The Nobel Prize is given every year in the six fields – literature, medicine, physics chemistry, peace and economics. The will of the Swedish inventor Alfred Nobel established the prizes in 1895. The prizes in five fields except economics were first awarded in 1901. The Nobel Memorial Prize in Economic Sciences was established by Sweden's central bank in 1968.

28. (b) Phycology is the scientific study of algae. Phycology or algology is a branch of life science and is often regarded as a sub-discipline of botany. It includes the study of prokary otic forms known as blue-green algae or cyanobacteria.

29. (a) King Camp Gillette, an American businessman, invented the best-selling version of the safety razor in 1901. Several models were in existence before Gillette' design. Gillette's innovation was the thin, inexpensive, disposable blade of stamped steel. Gillntte's is widely credited with inventing the so-called razor and blade's business model.

30. (d) Barter is a system of exchange where goods or services are directly exchanged for other goods or services without using a medium of exchange, such as money. Barter, as a replacement for money as the method of exchange, is used in times of monetary crisis, such as when the currency may be either unstable or simply unavailable for conducting commerce.

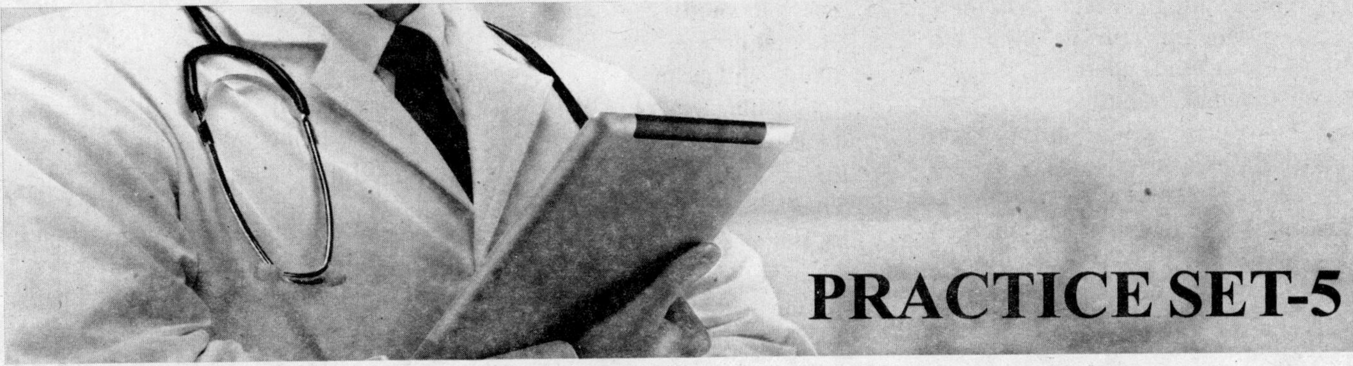

1. Vardhamana Mahavira attained Parinirvana at
(a) Saranath
(b) Pava
(c) Vaishali
(d) Shravanabelagola

2. Name the person who started 'Young Italy'.
(a) Garibaldi
(b) Joseph Mazzini
(c) Count Cavour
(d) Victor Emanuel

3. In which language did Babur write his memoirs called 'Tuzuk-i-Baburi'?
(a) Persian (b) Arabic
(c) Mongol (d) Turkish

4. The number of days for a year in Mercury is
(a) 56 (b) 88
(c) 36 (d) 300

5. The twin planet of the earth which resembles in size, density and mass is
(a) Mercury (b) Venus
(c) Mars (d) Jupiter

6. Lichens developing on rocky substrates are called
(a) Lignicolous
(b) Corticolous
(c) Saxicolous
(d) Terricolous

7. Heterothallism was discovered by
(a) E. J. Butler
(b) J. H. Gralgie
(c) A.F. Blakelee
(d) B.B. Mundkar

8. In the Sun, heat and light are produced by
(a) Chemical reactions
(b) Nuclear reactions
(c) Ionic reactions
(d) Biological reactions

9. The conductivity of a superconductor is
(a) Infinite (b) Large
(c) Small (d) Zero

10. Sodium chloride or table salt occurs in nature as the mineral
(a) Talc (b) Halite
(c) Sphalerite (d) Sylvlite

11. Which one of the following gases has colour?
(a) Chlorine (b) Hydrogen
(c) Nitrogen (d) Oxygen

12. The chemical name of Baking soda is
(a) Sodium hydroxide
(b) Sodium carbonate
(c) Sodium bicarbonate
(d) Sodium acetate

13. Nagarjuna Sagar project is on the river
(a) Sutlej (b) Narmada
(c) Krishna (d) Kaveri

14. State with highest percentage of forests is
(a) Arunachal Pradesh
(b) Mizoram
(c) Assam
(d) Uttar Pradesh

15. A.P.J. Abdul Kalam, the former president of India, is the author of the book
(a) The Wings of Fire and Ignited Minds
(b) The Algebra of Infinite Justice
(c) Four Fires and Death of Fire
(d) None of these

16. Which famous scientist was the first to look at the night sky through a telesçope?
(a) Galileo
(b) Copernicus
(c) Michael Faraday
(d) Newton

17. May 8 is observed as
(a) World Red Cross Day
(b) World Standard Day
(c) World Telecommunication Day
(d) Commonwealth Day

18. Mohiniattam dance form developed originally in which of the following states?
(a) Karnataka (b) Odisha
(c) Tamil Nadu (d) Kerala

19. Who is called the 'Grand Old Man' of India?
(a) Jawaharlal Nehru
(b) Dadabhai Naoroji
(c) Gopal Krishna Gokhale
(d) Mahatma Gandhi

20. Which of the following is used as raw material for the manufacture of rayon?
(a) Coal (b) Plastic
(c) Cellulose (d) Petroleum

21. The Vice President of India may be impeached by
(a) Lok Sabha
(b) Rajya Sabha
(c) Vidhan Sabha
(d) Vidhan Parishad

22. Which State Legislative Assembly has the maximum strength (number of members)?
(a) Andhra Pradesh
(b) West Bengal
(c) Maharashtra
(d) Uttar Pradesh

23. How many languages are there in the Eighth Schedule of the Constitution of India?
(a) 18 (b) 19
(c) 16 (d) 22

24. Who was the first speaker of free India?
(a) G.V. Mavalankar
(b) K.M. Munshi
(c) Frank Anthony
(d) Smt. Sarojini Naidu

25. The Lakshadweep Islands are situated in the
(a) Indian Ocean
(b) Arabian Sea
(c) Bay of Bengal
(d) None of these

26. The concept of Concurrent List in the Indian Constitution is borrowed from the Constitution of
(a) Japan (b) Canada
(c) Australia (d) USA

27. Inflation is caused by
(a) increase in money supply and decrease in production
(b) increase in money supply
(c) increase in production
(d) decrease in production

28. Which one of the following inscriptions relates to the Chalukya king, Pulakesin II?
(a) Maski
(b) Hathigumpha
(c) Aihole
(d) Nasik

29. Who among the following introduced the Mansabdari System?
(a) Shah Jahan (b) Sher Shah
(c) Akbar (d) Jahangir

30. Under which Article of the Constitution can an individual move to the Supreme Court directly in case of any violation of Fundamental Rights?
(a) Article 32 (b) Article 28
(c) Article 29 (d) Article 31

Answers with Explanations

1. (b) Vardhamana Mahavira attained parinirvana at the dawn of a no moon day at Pavapuri in Bihar when he was 72 years old (527 B.C). His nirvana is mentioned into the sacred text Kalpasutra. Pavapuri was the place where Mahavira gave his last discourse before death.

2. (b) Young Italy was a political movement founded in 1831 by Giuseppe Mazzini. The goal of this movement was to create a united Italian republic through promoting a general insurrection in the Italian reactionary states and in the lands occupied by the Austrian Empire.

3. (d) Tuzuk-i-Baburi (Letters of Babur) is an autobiographical work of Babur written in the Chagatal or Turkish language which was his native tongue. Turki or Turkish was the spoken language of the Andijan- Timurids. The book is also known as Babumama.

4. (b) Mercury orbits the sun once in every 88 Earth days. So one year on Mercury is 88 Earth days. Mercury is the closest planet to the sun. But a day on Mercury is longer than an Earth day; One Mercury day lasts for 59 Earth days. On average, it is a little more than one-third the distance from the sun than Earth is.

5. (b) Venus is sometimes called Earth's twin because Venus and Earth are almost the same size, have about the same mass, and have a very similar composition. They are also neighbouring planets. However, according to recent NASA reports, a new planet, named Kepler 452b, is "the closest twin to Earth."

6. (c) Lichen communities developed on rocky substratum are called as Saxicolous. The type of rock and pH are important factor responsible for colonization of the rock by lichen communities. The species like Caloplecta, Aspicilia grow on hard lime stones; Verrucaria species can be seen on well lit areas; Lepraria, Cystocoleus community grows on siliceous rocks.

7. (c) The term heterothallism was first used by Blakeslee in 1904. Heterothallic species have sexes that reside in different individuals. The term is applied particularly to distinguish heterothallic fungi, which require two compatible partners to produce sexual spores, from homothallic ones, which are capable of sexual reproduction from a single organism.

8. (b) The thermonuclear process of nuclear fusion releases an incredible amount of energy in the form of light and heat in the Sun. The core is the only region in the Sun that produces an appreciable amount of thermal energy through fusion. It is here, in the core, where energy is produced by hydrogen atoms (H) being converted into molecules of helium (He).

9. (a) Superconductors are materials that conduct electricity with no resistance. This means a superconductor can carry a current indefinitely without losing any energy. So a superconductor has the property of being a perfect conductor, or having infinite conductivity, or zero resistance. Resistivity is the reciprocal of conductivity,

10. (b) Sodium chloride (NaCl), also known as Common Salt, occurs in nature in cubic crystals of rock salt or halite. Halite are evaporite deposits formed by the evaporation of saline water in partially enclosed basins. They are characteristically associated with beds of limestone, dolomite, and shale.

11. (a) Chlorine is a yellow-green gas under standard conditions, where it forms diatomic molecules. It has a distinctive strong odor, familiar to most from common household bleach. Chlorine is an element of the halogen group. It has the highest electron affinity and the third highest electronegativity of all the reactive elements.

12. (c) Sodium bicarbonate ($NaHCO_3$) is known as baking soda. It is a salt composed of sodium ions and bicarbonate ions. Baking soda is primarily used in baking, as a leavening agent. It reacts with acidic components, releasing carbon dioxide, which causes expansion of the batter and forms the characteristic texture and grain in pancakes, cakes, quick breads, etc.

13. (c) Nagarjuna Sagar Dam is built across the Krishna river at Nagarjuna Sagar where the river forms boundary between Nalgonda district of Telangana state and Guntur district of Andhra Pradesh. It is one of the earliest multi-purpose irrigation and hydro-electric projects in India.

14. (b) As per the India State Forest Report 2015, among all the states and Union Territories, Mizoram has the highest forest cover with 88.93 percent of the total area, followed by Lakshadweep. The total forest and tree cover of India is 79.42 million hectare, which is 24.16 percent of its total geogra-phical area.

15. (a) Wings of Fire: An Auto-biography of A.P.J. Abdul Kalam (1999) is an autobio-graphy of A.P.J. Abdul Kalam, former President of India. He also authored Ignited Minds-Unleashing the Power Within India' (2002). Ignited Minds is a logical step forward from his earlier book, 'India 2020: A Vision for the New Millennium.'

16. (a) The science of astronomy took a huge leap forward in the first decade of the 1600s with the invention of the optical telescope and its use to study the night sky. Galileo Galilei did not invent the telescope but was the first to use it in 1609 for viewing Moon, Jupiter and the Milky Way. The basic tool that Galileo used was a crude refracting telescope.

17. (a) World Red Cross Red Crescent Day is celebrated on 8 May each year. This date is the anniversary of the birth of Henry Dunant, the founder of In ternational Committee of the Red Cross (ICRC) and the recipient of the first Nobel Peace Prize. The first Red Cross Day was celebrated on 8 May 1948.

18. (d) Mohiniattam is a classical dance form from Kerala, India. Believed to have originated in 16th century CE, it is one of the eight Indian classical dance forms recognized by the Sangeet Natak Akademi. It is a very graceful form of dance performed as solo recitals by women.

19. (b) Dadabhai Naoroji is known as the "Grand Old Man of India" and the "Father of Indian Nationalism". He played a key role in founding the Indian National Congress in 1885 along with A.O. Hume and D.E. Wacha. His book Poverty and Un-British Rule in India brought attention to the draining of India's wealth into Britain.

20. (c) Rayon is a manufactured regenerated cellulose fiber. It is made from purified cellulose, primarily from wood pulp, which is chemically converted into a soluble compound. Because rayon is manu-factured from naturally occurring polymers, it is considered as semi-synthetic fiber.

21. (b) The Vice-President cannot be formally impeached, unlike the President. The Constitution states that the Vice-President can be removed by a resolution of the Rajya Sabha passed by an effective majority (more than 50% of effective membership (total membership–vacant seats) and agreed to by a simple majority (50% of present and voting members) of the Lok Sabha (Article 67(b)).

22. (d) Uttar Pradesh with 404 legislative assembly seats has the highest number of seats. Before the reorganization of the State on 9 November 2000, the strength of the UP Legislative Assembly was 426. The strength of West Bengal Assembly is 295; Maharashtra: 288; Andhra Pradesh: 195.

23. (d) The Eighth Schedule to the Indian Constitution contains a list of 22 scheduled languages. Via the 92nd Constitutional amendment 2003, four new languages— Dogri, Maithili, Santali and Bodo were added to the 8th Schedule of the Indian Constitution.

24. (a) Ganesh Vasudev Mavalankar was the first Speaker of the Lok Sabha from 15 May 1952 to 13 January 1956. Earlier, he was the President of the Central Legislative Assembly (from 1946 to 1947), then Speaker of the Constituent Assembly of India.

25 . (b) Lakshadweep is an archipelago of islands in the Laccadive Sea, part of the Arabian Sea. It lies off the south-western coast of India. The archipelago comprises of 36 main islands, many smaller islands, coral atolls and coral reefs. Lakshadweep is recognized as the smallest union territory of India.

26. (c) The Indian Constitution borrowed the concept of concurrent list from Australia. From the Australian Constitution, India also borrowed the features of Freedom of Trade, Commerce and Inter State Trade, and Joint Sitting in the Parliament.

27. (a) Economists generally agree that in the long run, inflation is caused by increase in the money supply. According to the theory of Demand-Pull

Inflation, if demand grows faster than supply, prices will increase. There is too much money chasing too few goods. The increase in money supply is not matched by the equivalent production of goods.

28. (c) The Aihole inscriptions were written by Ravikirti, court poet of Chalukya King, Pulakesin II, who reigned from 610 CE to 642 CE. This inscription gives information about the conquests of Pulakesin, especially how he defeated Harshavardhana.

29. (c) The Mansabdari system introduced by Akbar was a unique feature of the administrative system of the Mughal Empire. It was a system common to both the military and the civil department. The term is derived from Mansab, meaning 'rank'. Hence, Mansabdar literally means 'rank-holder'.

30. (a) Right to Constitutional remedies under Article 32 of the Indian Constitution empowers the citizens to move to a court of law in case of any denial of the fundamental rights. The courts can issue various kinds of writs, such as habeas corpus, mandamus, prohibition, quo warranto and certiorari.

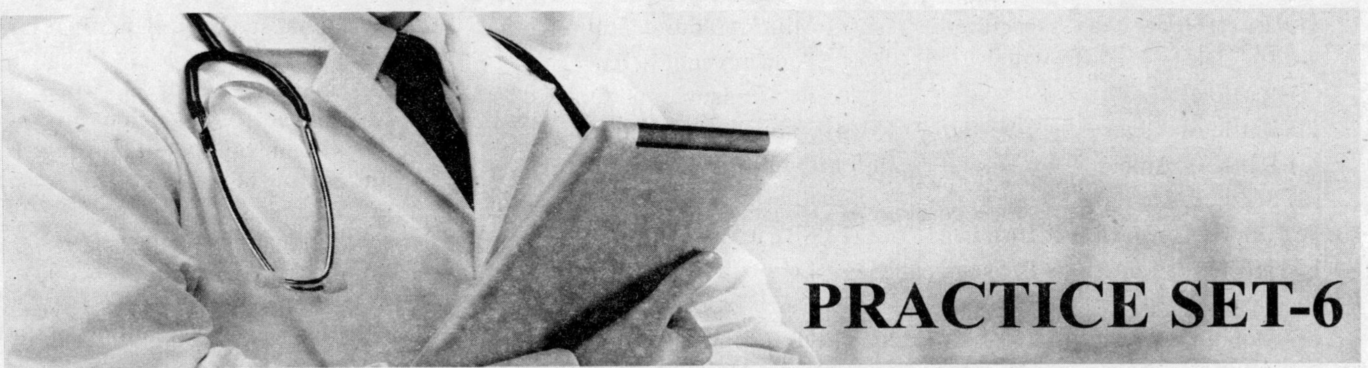

PRACTICE SET-6

1. **Which blood vessels carry pure blood from the lungs to the heart?**
(a) Pulmonary arteries
(b) Pulmonary veins
(c) Cardiac artery
(d) Cardiac vein
2. **Kala-azar is transmitted by**
(a) Sand fly (b) Tsetse fly
(c) Black flies (d) Mites
3. **Which of the following units used to measure the speed of a computer?**
(a) SYPS (b) MIPS
(c) BAUD (d) Byte
4. **The chemical name of quick lime is**
(a) Calcium hydroxide
(b) Calcium oxide
(c) Calcium chloride
(d) Calcium carbonate
5. **Which of the following are used to prepare the main storage (starch) form of food in plants?**
(a) Carbon dioxide and oxygen
(b) Water and oxygen
(c) Carbon dioxide and nitrogen
(d) Carbon dioxide and water
6. **The antacid marketed as milk of magnesia has as main in gredient :**
(a) $MgCO_3$ (b) $MgSO_4$
(c) $Mg(OH)_2$ (d) $MgCl_2$
7. **Presence of excess fluorine in water causes.**
(a) Fluorosis
(b) Dental Cavity
(c) Tooth Decay
(d) Respiratory disease
8. **The largest tea growing country in the World is**
(a) Sri Lanka (b) China
(c) India (d) Brazil
9. **The first person ever to reach the South Pole was**
(a) Amundsen
(b) Peary
(c) Magellan
(d) Amerigo Vespucci
10. **Who amongst the following is the author of the book 'Name Sake'?**
(a) Vikram Seth
(b) Jhumpa Lahiri
(c) Kiran Desai
(d) Shobha De
11. **National Science Day is observed on**
(a) 5th January
(b) 28th February
(c) 14th March
(d) 2nd June
12. **The largest proven oil reserve of the world lies in**
(a) Venezuela (b) Saudi Arabia
(c) Iran (d) Iraq
13. **The book 'Gokhale, My Political Guru' was written by**
(a) M.A. Jinnah (b) M.K. Gandhi
(c) Shaukat Ali (d) C.R. Das
14. **Kudankulam Project is located in which state?**
(a) Karnataka (b) Tamil Nadu
(c) Telangana (d) Kerala
15. **Who was the first black actor to win Oscar?**
(a) Eddie Murphy
(b) Wesley Snipes
(c) Sidney Poitiers
(d) Morgan Freeman
16. **The original name of 'Mahabharata' is**
(a) Kathasarıtsagar
(b) Jai Samhita
(c) Rajtarangini
(d) Bharat Katha
17. **Who fixes the REPO rate in India?**
(a) RBI (Reserve Bank of India)
(b) IMF (International Monetary Fund)
(c) WTO (World Trade Organization)
(d) SEBI (Securities and Exchange Board of India)
18. **An indirect instrument of monetary policy is**
(a) Bank rate
(b) Cash reserve ratio
(c) Open market operations
(d) Statutory liquidity ratio
19. **Who first gave the concept of "Distributive Justice"?**
(a) Plato (b) Aristotle
(c) Machiavelli (d) Locke
20. **The reorganization of states on linguistic basis was done in**
(a) 1950 (b) 1951
(c) 1952 (d) 1956
21. **Who among the following was responsible for the founding of the Muhammadan Alglo-Oriental College?**
(a) Sir Sayyid Ahmad Khan
(b) Yusuf Ali
(c) Muhammad Iqbal
(d) Altaf Husain

22. Sir Eyre Coote was associated with which of the following?
(a) Battle of Wandiwash
(b) Battle of Adyar
(c) Battle of Ambur
(d) Seize of Arcot

23. Which among the following inscription is known as Prayaga Prashasti?
(a) Mehrauli Inscription
(b) Allahabad Pillar Inscription
(c) Hathigumpha Inscription
(d) Aihole Inscription

24. Which among the following is related to Sadr-us-Sadr?
(a) Military administration
(b) Land revenue
(c) Ecclesiastical matters
(d) Judicial administration

25. Philadelphia is famous for
(a) Ship-building
(b) Silk textiles
(c) Locomotives
(d) Dairy industry

26. The Dandi March of Gandhiji is an example of
(a) Direct Action
(b) Boycott
(c) Civil Disobedience
(d) Non-Cooperation

27. The longest river of peninsular India is
(a) Krishna (b) Kaveri
(c) Narmada (d) Godavari

28. The Himalayan mountain range is an example of
(a) Volcanic mountain
(b) Residual mountain
(c) Block mountain
(d) Fold mountain

29. A cellulosic wall is found in the cells of
(a) animals (b) bacteria
(c) fungi (d) plants

30. The filtration unit of kidney is
(a) axon (b) nephron
(c) neuron (d) yellow fibre

Answers with Explanations

1. (b) The pulmonary veins are large blood vessels that receive oxygenated blood from the lungs and drain into the left atrium of the heart. There are four pulmonary veins, two from each lung. They play an essential role in respiration, by receiving blood that has been oxygenated in the alveoli.

2. (a) Kala-azar, the most severe form of leishmaniasis, is a parasitic disease transmitted by the bite of infected female sandflies. Sandfly of genus Phlebotomus argentipes are the only known vectors of kala-azar in India. Kala-azar is also known as black fever, and Dumdum fever.

3. (b) MIPS (Million Instructions Per Second) is a unit for measuring computer speed. The number of MIPS (million instructions per second) is a general measure of computing performance and, by implication, the amount of work a larger computer can do.

4. (b) Calcium oxide (CaO) is commonly known as quicklime or burnt lime. It is usually made by the thermal decomposition of materials such as limestone, or seashells, that contain calcium carbonate ($CaCO_3$) in a lime kiln. It is a key ingredient for the process of making cement.

5. (d) Plants synthesize food directly from carbon dioxide and water using energy of light. In photosynthesis, chlorophyll in the leaves of plants absorbs light energy from the Sun. Plants use this energy to convert water and CO_2 from the environment into glucose and oxygen.

$$6CO_2 + 6H_2O \xrightarrow{\text{Sunlight energy}} C_6H_{12}O_6 + 6O_2$$

6. (c) Magnesium hydroxide $Mg(OH)_2$ is often known as milk of magnesia, because of its milk-like appearance as a suspension. It is a common component of antacids and laxatives since it interferes with the absorption of folic acid and iron. The antacid properties come from the hydroxide ions which are responsible for neutralizing the acid.

7. (a) Fluorosis is a disease caused by water that contains high amount of fluoride and particularly in groundwater. It leads to hypomineralization of tooth enamel caused by ingestion of excessive fluoride during enamel formation. A major cause of fluorosis is the inappropriate use of fluoride-containing dental products such as toothpaste and mouth rinses.

8. (b) China is the largest producer of tea in the world. It contributes about 30-35 percent of the global tea production. India and Kenya come at second and third positions. Several varieties are produced in China including green, oolong, white, pu-erh, and jasmine teas to name a few.

9. (a) Roald Amundsen was a Norwegian explorer who led the Antarctic expedition of 1910-12 he was the first to reach the South Pole, on 14 December 1911. In 1926, he was the first expedition leader for the air expedition to the North Pole.

10. (b) The Namesake (2004) is the first novel by Jhumpa Lahiri. It was originally a novella published in The New Yorker and was later expanded to a full-length novel. The novel describes the struggles and hardships of a Bengali couple who immigrate to the United States to form a life outside of everything they are accustomed to.

11. (b) National Science Day is celebrated in India on 28 February each year to mark the discovery of the Raman effect by Indian physicist Sir C.V. Raman on 28 February 1928. For his discovery, Raman was awarded the Nobel Prize in Physics in 1930.

12. (a) Based on data from OPEC at the beginning of 2013, the highest proved oil reserves including non-conventional oil deposits are in Venezuela (20% of global reserves), Saudi Arabia (18% of global reserves), Canada (13% of global reserves), and Iran (9%).

13. (b) "Gokhale - My political guru" has been authored by Mohandas Karamchand Gandhi. It is a small book of 60 pages that was published in 1955. This book is compilation of Gandhi's writings and speeches on Gokhale, mostly in Gujarati.

14. (b) Kudankulam Nuclear Power Plant is a nuclear power station in Kudankulam in the Tirunelveli district of Tamil Nadu. It is a joint Russia-India project. Construction on the plant began on 31 March 2002, but faced several delays due to the fishermen's objection.

15. (c) Sidney Poitier won the best actor Oscar for his role in 'Lilies of the Field' in 1963, becoming the first black actor to win the award. Besides Vie was the first Bahamian to win an Oscar award. The film was adapted by James Poe from the 1962 novel of the same name by William Edmund Barrett. It was produced and directed by Ralph Nelson.

16. (b) The original name of Mahabharata was "Jaya Samhita" as coined by Vyasa. When first narrated, it had only 8,800 shlokas and its original name was "Jaya" as written by Ganesha. The full 100,000 verses of the book was completed several centuries later by addition of many stories and was finally named as 'Mahabharata'.

17. (a) Repo rate is the rate at which the central bank of a country lends money to commercial banks in the event of any shortfall of funds. In India, it is set by the Reserve Bank of India. Repo rate is used by monetary authorities to control inflation.

18. (c) The indirect or market based instruments of monetary policy comprise open market operations and the use of 'Repo' rate. An open market operation involves buying or selling of government securities from or to the public and banks. The RBI sells government securities to control the flow of credit and buys government securities to increase credit flow.

19. (b) An early theory of justice was set out by the Ancient Greek philosopher Plato in his work The Republic. Aristotle developed it into his concept of Distributive Justice. Aristotle's Distributive Justice is the name of that principle of distribution by which goods, services, honour and offices are distributed among the citizens of the state. It is the other name of proportionate equality.

20. (d) The states were reorganized on the basis of language in 1956 under the States Reorganisation Act. On the basis of linguistic considerations, India was divided into 14 states and 6 union territories under the States Reorganization Act 1956.

21. (a) The Mohammedan Anglo-Oriental College was established by Sir Syed Ahmad Khan in 1875. It became Aligarh Muslim University in 1920. Sir Mohammad Ali Mohammad Khan and the Aga Khan III also played a major role in its establishment.

22. (a) Eyre Coote was a Lieutenant General in the British Army in India who won the Battle of Wandiwash against the French in 1760. His victory at the Battle of Wandiwash is considered a decisive turning point in the struggle for control in India between Britain and France.

23. (a) Prayag-Prasasti is also known as Allahabad Pillar inscription. Composed by Harisena, this inscription talks about the achievements of Samudragupta. It is considered the most important historical document of the classical Gupta age. It is in Sanskrit.

24. (c) Sadr-us-Sudur was the head of public charities and ecclesiastical department. He was the head of the religious department. His primary duties were the propagation of Islam, observance of its principles and protection of the privileges of Muslims.

25. (c) Building of locomotives is the most famous manufacturing business of Philadelphia in USA. It is known for Baldwin Locomotive Works which dominated the locomotive industry since the 20th century. It was once known as the Workshop to the world.

26. (a) The Salt March which began with the Dandi March on 12th March, 1930 was an important part of the Indian independence movement. It was a direct action campaign of tax resistance and non-violent protest against the British salt monopoly in colonial India.

27. (d) The Godavari (1450 km) is the longest river of peninsular India, followed by Krishna (about 1300 km). It has the second largest river basin in India after the Ganges. It is often referred to as the Vridha (Old) Ganga or the Dakshina (South) Ganga.

28. (d) The Himalayas are among the youngest mountain ranges on the planet and consist mostly of uplifted sedimentary and metamorphic rock. They are Fold Mountains which were formed due to a continental collision or orogeny along the convergent boundary between the Indo-Australian Plate and the Eurasian Plate.

29. (d) Cellulose is an important structural component of the primary cell wall of green plants, many forms of algae and the oomycetes. It is a complex carbohydrate, $(C_6H_{10}O_5)$, that is composed of glucose units.

30. (b) Nephron is the basic structural and functional unit of the kidney. Its chief function is to regulate the concentration of water and soluble substances like sodium salts by filtering the blood, reabsorbing what is needed and excreting the rest as urine.

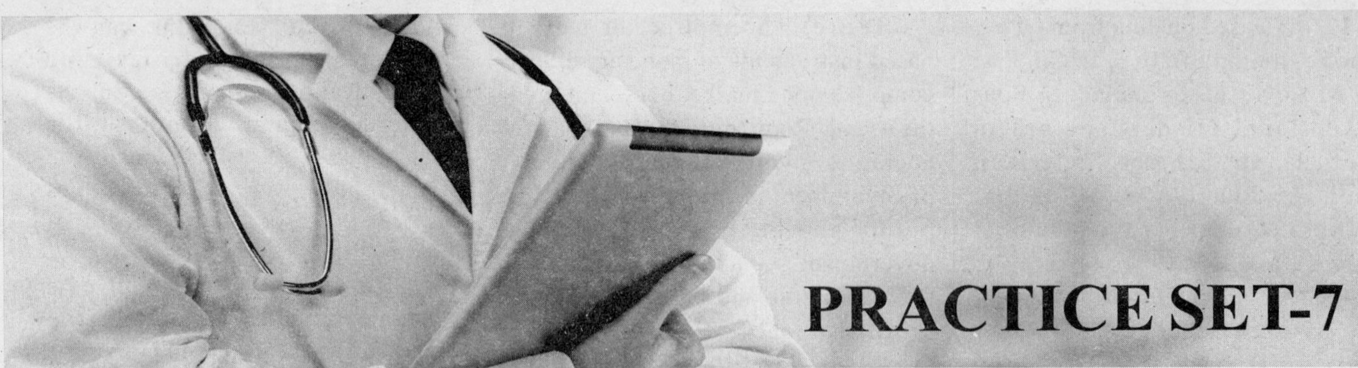

PRACTICE SET-7

1. A Trade Cycle consists of
(a) Three Phases (b) Four Phases
(c) Five Phases (d) Six Phases

2. The Khilafat Movement was organized to protest against
(a) religious interference by the British
(b) Russian Revolution
(c) dismemberment of Turkey
(d) suppression of Pathans

3. Planning Commission was established in the year
(a) 1980 (b) 1970
(c) 1950 (d) 1960

4. India witnessed single party domination till
(a) 1962 (b) 1967
(c) 1971 (d) 1977

5. Which part of the Constitution of India has been described as the soul of the Constitution ?
(a) Fundamental Rights
(b) Directive Principles of State Policy
(c) Preamble
(d) Panchayats.

6. Constituent Assembly adopted the Constitution on
(a) 15th August 1947
(b) 26th November 1949
(c) 26th January 1950
(d) 30th January 1948

7. The rustless Iron Pillar at Mehrauli (Delhi) was erected by the
(a) Mauryas
(b) Kushans
(c) Guptas
(d) Satavahanas

8. The famous 'Gayatri Mantra' has been taken from
(a) Rigveda (b) Samaveda
(c) Yajurveda (d) Atharvaveda

9. The Rajput King who was defeated by Babur in the battle of Khanwa was
(a) Udai Singh
(b) Rana Pratap Singh
(c) Rana Sanga
(d) Rudra Deva

10. Who was the founder of the Ramakrishna Mission ?
(a) Sri Ramakrishna
(b) Swami Shraddhananda
(c) Keshab Chandra
(d) Swami Vivekananda

11. Who led the Mutiny at Kanpur?
(a) Begum Hazrat Mahal
(b) Nana Sahib
(c) Tantla Tope
(d) Rani Laxmlbal

12. Which 'Water Body' separates Andaman and Nicobar Islands?
(a) Andaman Sea
(b) Bay of Bengal
(c) Ten Degree Channel
(d) Eleventh Degree Channel

13. State Highways are maintained by
(a) Individual States
(b) Central Government
(c) Central and State Governments jointly
(d) Private parties selected by the State Governments

14. The first port developed after Independence was
(a) Nhava Sheva
(b) Kandla
(c) New Mangalore
(d) Mumbai

15. The neighbouring country of India which has the smallest area is
(a) Sri Lanka (b) Bangladesh
(c) Bhutan (d) Nepal

16. Kaziranga Wild Life Sanctuary is in the State of
(a) Bihar (b) Tamil Nadu
(c) Assam (d) Kerala

17. Resin is extracted from
(a) Papaya (b) Pine
(c) Rubber (d) Banyan

18. A common plant found in tropical rainforest is
(a) Pine (b) Eucalyptus
(c) Orchid (d) Fir

19. Which of the following vitamins is necessary for clotting of blood?
(a) K (b) C
(c) A (d) B

20. Influenza virus contains
(a) RNA only
(b) DNA only
(c) Both RNA and DNA in equal proportion.
(d) DNA with very small proportion of RNA.

21. Lung fish is a link between
(a) Amphibia and Birds
(b) Reptiles and Birds
(c) Amphibia and Reptiles
(d) Reptiles and Mammals

22. Green gland is the excretory organ of
(a) Earthworm (b) Cockroach
(c) Prawn (d) House-fly

23. When pressure is increased, the boiling point of water
(a) decreases
(b) increases
(c) remains the same
(d) depends on the volume of vapour formed

24. In the treatment of skin disease the radio isotope used is
(a) Radio phosphorous
(b) Radio iodine
(c) Radio lead
(d) Radio cobalt

25. Rainbow has : (Choose incorrect statement)
(a) red light as its outer-most colour towards sky
(b) red light as its inner-most colour towards earth
(c) violet light as its innermost colour towards earth
(d) its curvature bent towards earth.

26. Which Indian industry is employing large number of workers?
(a) Iron and Steel Industry
(b) Textile Industry
(c) Jute Industry
(d) Sugar Industry

27. To which category does right to vote belong?
(a) Human Rights
(b) Civil Rights
(c) Natural Rights
(d) Political Rights

28. Which dynasty immediately succeeded the Maurya dynasty and ruled Magadha Kingdom?
(a) Satvahana (b) Sunga
(c) Nanda (d) Kanva

29. How many members are nominated by the President to Rajya Sabha?
(a) 2 (b) 12
(c) 15 (d) 20

30. The Chairman of the Public Accounts Committee of the Parliament is appointed by
(a) Speaker of Lok Sabha
(b) Prime Minister of India
(c) President of India
(d) Chairman of Rajya Sabha

Answers with Explanations

1. (b) Trade cycle is more or less regular periods of increasing economic activity followed by periods of decreasing economic activity. It consists of four phases : Prosperity Phase, Recession Phase, Depression Phase and Recovery Phase.

2. (c) In support of the Khilafat movement Gandhiji inaugurated the Non-Cooperation campaign with a bang on August 1, 1920.

3. (c) Planning Commission was established in the form of an advisory and specialised institution in 1950.

4. (b) India witnessed single party domination till 1967.

5. (c) Preamble to the Constitution is soul of the Constitution.

6. (b) Constituent Assembly adopted the Constitution on November 26, 1949. From this date the provisions relating to citizenship, elections, provisional parliament, temporary and transitional provisions were given immediate effect. The rest of the Constitution came into effect on January 26, 1950 which is referred to in the Constitution as the Date of its Commencement.

7. (c) It is believed that the rustless Iron Pillar at Mehrauli in Delhi was erected by the Gupta ruler.

8. (a) The famous "Gayatri Mantra' has been taken from Rig Veda. Rig Veda consists of 1017 hymns and is divided into 10 mandalas.

9. (c) Babur defeated Rana Sanga in the Battle of Khanwa in 1527 AD.

10. (d) Swami Vivekananda founded the Ramakrishna Mission in Belur in 1897.

11. (b) Nana Sahib was proclaimed the Peshwa. General Sir Hugh Wheeler, commanding the station, surrendered on June 27, 1857. At Kanpur, Nana Sahib was joined by his able and experienced Lieutenant Tantia Tope. Sir Campbell occupied Kanpur on December 6, 1857.

12. (c) Andaman and Nicobar Islands are separated by Ten Degree Channel.

13. (a) State Highways are the responsibility of state Government and are maintained through various agencies.

14. (b) The first port developed after Independence was Kandla. New Mangalore was declared a major port in 1974. Kandla was constructed in the 1950s as the chief sea port serving western India.

15. (c) Country Area : Sri Lanka : 65,610 sq.km, Bangladesh : 144,000 sq.km, Bhutan : 47,000 sq.km, Nepal : 140,800 sq.km

16. (c) Kaziranga Wild Life Sanctuary is in the State of Assam. It is famous for one-horned Great Indian Rhinoceros.

17. (b) Resin is extracted from fir or pine. It is an adhesive inflammable substance insoluble in water.

18. (c) Orchid, mahogny rosewood, cincona etc. are found in Tropical Rainforest.

19. (a) Vitamin K is necessary for clotting of blood. It was discovered by Dam and Doisy of United States in 1935.

20. (a) Influenza virus has a layer of spikes on the outside. Inside the layer of spikes, there are eight pieces of RNA.

21. (c)

22. (c) Green gland is excretory organ of some crustaceans, like prawn.

23. (b) When pressure is increased, the boiling point of water increases. At 16 bar, the boiling point of water is 200°C.

24. (a) Radio phosphorus is used in the treatment of leukaemia.

Radio iodine— thyroid disorders.

25. (b) Red colour appears on the upper side of a rainbow and violet colour on the lower side. Option (b) is incorrect.

26. (a) Workers in the iron and steel industry hold more than 2000 different types of jobs. About 80 % of all the workers are directly engaged in moving raw materials and steel products from and to the plants, making iron and steel products, and maintaining the vast amount of machinery used in the industry. In addition, other workers are needed to do clerical, sales, professional, technical, administrative and supervisory works.

27. (d) Political participation is the basis of democracy and a vital part of the enjoyment of all human rights. The right of all people to vote in elections, without any discrimination, is one of the most fundamental of all human rights and civil liberties. However, since democracy is in itself a political process, Right to Vote should be counted as a fundamental political right as it is preservative of all rights.

28. (b) The Sunga Dynasty was established by Pusyamitra Sunga, after the fall of the Mauryan Empire. The last Mauryan emperor Brihadratha was assassinated by the then commander-in-chief of the Mauryan armed forces, Pusyamitra Sunga in 185 B.C.

29. (b) 12 members are nominated by the President to the Rajya Sabha. These members are nominated on the basis of their contributions to art, literature, science, and social services.

30. (a) The Chairman of the Public Accounts Committee (PAC) is appointed by the Speaker of the Lok Sabha. Since 1967, the chairman of the committee is selected from the opposition. The term of office of the members is one year.

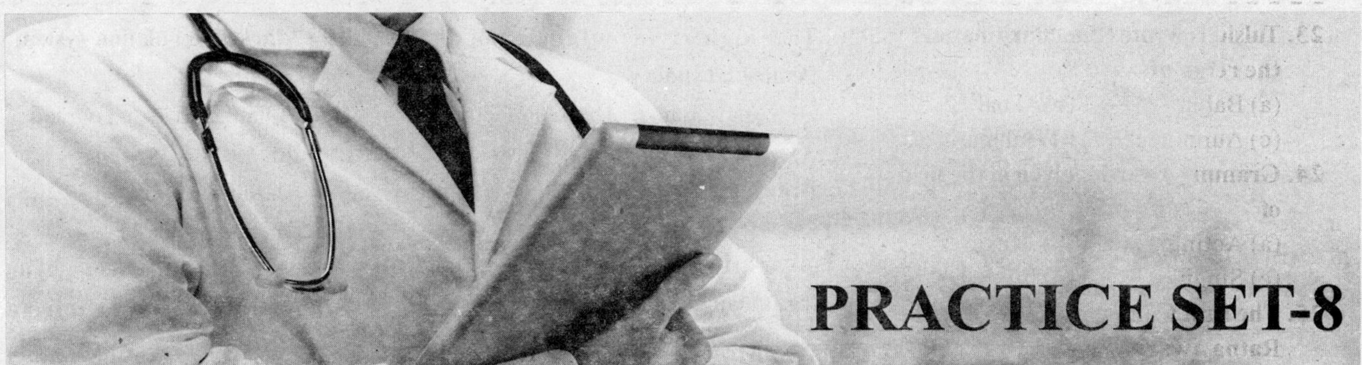

PRACTICE SET-8

1. Which of the following are consumer semi-durable goods?

(a) Cars and television sets
(b) Milk and Milk products
(c) Foodgrains and other food products
(d) Electrical appliance like fans and electric irons.

2. In which year were the States recognized on linguistic basis?

(a) 1951 (b) 1947
(c) 1950 (d) 1956

3. Who has got the power to create All India Services?

(a) Supreme Court
(b) The Parliament
(c) Council of Ministers
(d) Prime Minister

4. The "Mein Kampf" was written by

(a) Hitler (b) Mussolini
(c) Bismarck (d) Mazzini

5. When did the reign of Delhi Sultanate came to end ?

(a) 1498 A.D. (b) 1526 A.D.
(c) 1565 A.D. (d) 1600 A.D.

6. Who admits a new State to the Union of India ?

(a) President
(b) Supreme Court
(c) Prime Minister
(d) Parliament

7. India is the largest producer and exporter of

(a) Cotton (b) Copper
(c) Tea (d) Mica

8. The soils which are rich in Calcium are known as

(a) Pedocals (b) Pedalfers
(c) Podsols (d) Laterites

9. From which part of Opium plant we get morphine ?

(a) Leaves (b) Stem
(c) Bark (d) Fruit coat

10. Which of the following is a Biological method of soil conservations ?

(a) Contour farming
(b) Contour terracing
(c) Gully control
(d) Basin listing

11. Glucose is a type of

(a) Pentose sugar
(b) Hexose sugar
(c) Tetrose sugar
(d) Diose sugar

12. The original founder of the Manuscripts and Editor of Kautilya's Arthashastra was

(a) Srikanta Shastri
(b) Srinivasa Iyangar
(c) R. Shamashastri
(d) William Jones

13. Which of the following is the largest Biosphere Reserves of India ?

(a) Nilgiri
(b) Nandadevi
(c) Sundarbans
(d) Gulf of Mannar

14. Golden view of sea shell is due to

(a) Diffraction
(b) Dispersion
(c) Polarization
(d) Reflection

15. An object covers distance which is directly proportional to the square of the time. Its accelaration is

(a) increasing (b) decreasing
(c) zero (d) constant

16. Which of the following metals has least melting point ?

(a) Gold (b) Silver
(c) Mercury (d) Copper

17. The gas produced in marshy places due to decomposition of vegetation is

(a) Carbon monoxide
(b) Carbon dioxide
(c) Sulphur dioxide
(d) Methane

18. In cactus, the spines are the modified

(a) stem (b) stipulse
(c) leaves (d) buds

19. Rainbow is formed due to

(a) refraction and dispersion
(b) scattering and refraction
(c) diffraction and refraction
(d) refraction and reflection

20. The boiling point of water decreases at higher altitudes is due to

(a) low temperature
(b) low atmospheric pressure
(c) high temprature
(d) high atmospheric pressure

21. The chemical name of "Hypo" commonly used in photography is

(a) Sodium thiosulphate
(b) Silver nitrate
(c) Sodium nitrate
(d) Silver iodide

22. With what bio-region is the term "Steppe" associated ?

(a) Grasslands
(b) Tropical forests
(c) Savanna
(d) Coniferous forests

23. Tulsidas wrote Ramcharitmanas in the reign of
(a) Babur (b) Akbar
(c) Aurangzeb (d) Jahangir

24. Grammy Award is given in the field of
(a) Acting (b) Music
(c) Singing (d) Boxing

25. The first woman to get the Bharat Ratna Award is
(a) Mother Teresa
(b) Indira Gandhi
(c) Lata Mangeshkar
(d) Sarojini Naidu

26. The highest mountain peak in Peninsular India is
(a) Anaimudi (b) Dodabetta
(c) Mahendragiri (d) Nilgiris

27. Breaking down of rock *in situ* is known as
(a) erosion
(b) weathering
(c) mass wasting
(d) degradation

28. The longest river of Europe is
(a) Rhine (b) Rhone
(c) Danube (d) Volga

29. The Market Regulation system was introduced by
(a) Muhammad-Bin-Tughlaq
(b) Iltutmish
(c) Ala-ud-din Khilji
(d) Ghias-ud-din

30. Which of the following Mughal Emperors wrote their own autobiographies?
(a) Shah Alam and Farukh Siyar
(b) Babur and Jahangir
(c) Jahangir and Shah Jahan
(d) Akbar and Aurangzeb

Answers with Explanations

1. (c) Goods which are neither indestructible nor lasting are defined as semi durable goods. They fall in the category between durable goods and non durable goods. Some common semi durable goods are clothing or preserved foods; vehicles and electronic home appliances are classified as durable goods.

2. (d) Indian states were reorganized on 1 November 1956 under the States Reorganization Act, 1956. Andhra State was merged with the Telugu speaking area of Hyderabad state (also known as Telangana) to create Andhra Pradesh in 1956. Similarly Kerala in the south and three states (Uttar Pradesh, Bihar and Madhya Pradesh) came into being in the Hindi speaking area. West Bengal, Rajasthan, and Punjab were enlarged by addition of territories.

3. (b) Article 312 provides that an All India Service can be created only if the Council of States (Rajya Sabha) declares, by resolution supported by not less than two-thirds majority, that it is necessary in the national interest to create one or more such All India Services. When once such a resolution is passed, the Parliament is competent to constitute such an All India Service.

4. (a) Mein Kampf is an autobiographical manifesto by Nazi leader Adolf Hitler, in which he outlines his political ideology and future plans for Germany. Volume 1 of Mein Kampf was published in 1925 and Volume 2 in 1926. The book was edited by Rudolf Hess.

5. (b) The Delhi Sultanate ruled over large parts of India for 320 years from 1206 to 1526 A.D. The last ruler, Ibrahim Lodi, was defeated in the first Battle of Panipat (1526 A.D.) by Babur who laid the foundation of the Mughal Empire in India.

6. (d) Article 2 states that the parliament may, by law, admit new states into Union of India or establish new states on terms and conditions its deems fit. Article 3 empowers the parliament to form a new state by separation of a part of territory of an established state or to unite two or more states or parts of states or by uniting any territory to a part of any state.

7. (d) India is not only the largest producer but also the largest exporter of mica in the world. Andhra Pradesh is the largest producer of mica (Geography of India by Majid Hussain). It is the second largest producer and exporter of tea after China in the world.

8. (a) Pedocal soil is characterized by an abundance of calcium carbonate and calcium oxide. Pedocals are common in arid or semi arid regions where the rate of evaporation is greater than the rate of leaching. It has low soil organic matter.

9. (d) Morphine is the predominant alkaloid found in the varieties of opium poppy plant. It is obtained in form of liquid from the fruit capsule of the poppy. The latex which oozes from the incisions is collected and dried to produce "raw opium" (about 8-14% morphine by dryweight).

10. (a) The biological methods of soil conservation include contour farming, strip cropping. tillage operation, mulching, etc. Contour farming is practised in the hilly regions or on the slopes. The contours (circular or peripheral furrows) catch the downwardly moving water untilit is absorbed in the soil. It reduces run off, saves more water for crops, and reduces soil erosion.

11. (b) Three common sugars (glucose, galactose and fructose) share the same molecular formula: $C_6H_{12}O_6$. Because of their six carbon atoms, each is a hexose. They are "single" sugars or monosaccharides.

12. (c) In 1905, R. Ramashashtri discovered and published the Arthashastra, an ancient Indian treatise on statecraft. He transcribed, edited and published the Sanskrit edition in 1909. He proceeded to translate it into English, publishing it in 1915.

13. (d) The Gulf of Mannar located in Tamil Nadu is one of South Asia's largest biosphere reserves. It extends from Rameswaram Island in the North to Kanyakumari in the South of Tamil Nadu and Sri Lanka. It is spread over an area of 10,500 km^2. The area of other biosphere reserves (in km^2) is as follows: Sundarbans: 9630; Nilgiri: 5520; Nandadevi: 5860.

14. (c) When a ray of light falls on sea shell, its small amount gets refracted (slightly polarized) and rest almost gets reflected back (fully polarized). So it gets a golden view because of polarization.

15. (d) When an object covers distance which is directly proportional to the square of the time, its acceleration is constant. This is seen in the cases of falling objects. This connection between time and distance was first observed by Galileo.

16. (c) The melting point of the given metals (in Celsius) are: Gold: 1063; Silver: 961;Copper: 1083; Mercury:–38.86. Mercury is the only elemental metal known to melt at a generally cold temperature.

17. (d) Methane gas is a hydrocarbon gas largely composed of methane formed when organic material or vegetation decays in the absence of air. Naturally occurring methane is mainly produced by the process of methanogenesis. It is also known as Swamp Gas.

18. (c) Most cactus morphologists have concluded that cactus spines are modified leaves. They are wholly transformed leaves that protect the plant from herbivores, radiate heat from the stem during the day, and collect and drip condensed water vapour during the cooler night.

19. (d) A rainbow is an optical phenomenon that is caused by both reflection and refraction of light in water droplets resulting in a spectrum of light appearing in the sky. It is caused by light being refracted (bent) when entering a droplet of water, then reflected inside on the back of the droplet and refracted again when leaving it.

20. (b) At higher altitudes, the air pressure is decreased, which forces water's boiling point to lower. The air pressure decreases with altitude because of the decrease in the density of air. The lowered boiling point of water requires an increase incooking times or temperature.

21. (a) An emulsion of sodium thiosulfate is called hypo by photographers. It is used to stop development of exposed film. Thiosulfate converts undeveloped silver bromide grains in the film into water-soluble silver thiosulfate complexes that can be removed when the film is washed.

22. (a) The Steppe is a dry, cold, grassland that is found in all of the continents except Australia and Antarctica. It is mostly found in the USA, Mongolia, Siberia, Tibet and China, is usually found between the desert and the forest.

23. (b) Tulsidas wrote the Ramcharitmanas in Ayodhya in Vikram Samvat during the reign of Akbar (1556-1605 A.D.). It is an epic poem in Awadhi. Ramcharitmanas literally means "lake of the deeds of Rama".

24. (b) The Grammy Award is an accolade by the National Academy of Recording Arts and Sciences (NARAS) of the United States to recognize outstanding achievement in the music industry. The first Grammy Awards ceremony was held on May 4, 1959.

25. (b) Indira Gandhi became the first woman to receive the Bharat Ratna in 1971. She served as the Prime Minister of India from 1966 to 1977 and then again from 1980 until her assassination in 1984. Instituted in 1954, the Bharat Ratna is the highest civilian award of India.

26. (a) The highest peak of Peninsular India is Anaimudi (2695 m) in Anaimalai Hills. It is located in Kerala in the Western Ghats.

27. (b) Weathering is the breaking down of rocks, soils and minerals as well as artificial materials through contact with the Earth's atmosphere, biota and waters. Weathering occurs in situated or with no movement.

28. (d) The Volga is the largest river in Europe in terms of length, discharge, and watershed. It flows through the western part of Russia, and is widely viewed as the national river of Russia.

29. (c) Alauddin Khilji's measures to control the markets were one of the most important policy initiatives. Since Alauddin wanted to maintain a large army, he, therefore, lowered and fixed the price of the commodities of daily use.

30 . (b) Babur wrote his memoirs which form the main source for details of his life. They are known as the Baburnama. Jahangir, too, wrote his autobiography titlad 'Tuzuki Jahangiri'.

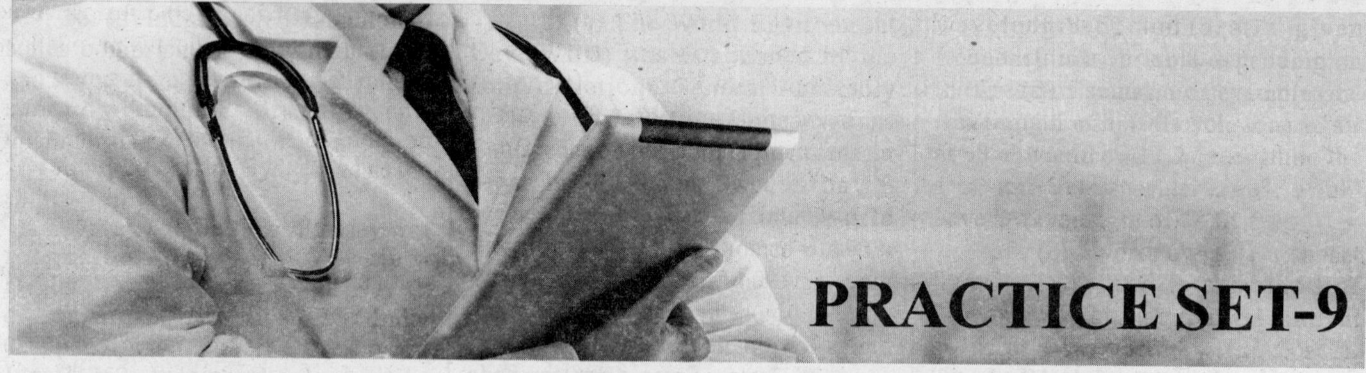

PRACTICE SET-9

1. **The terms 'Bull' and 'Bear' are associated with**
   (a) Banking
   (b) Foreign Trade
   (c) Stock Market
   (d) Internet Trade
2. **A currency whose exchange rate is influenced by the government is a/an**
   (a) Unmanaged Currency
   (b) Managed Currency
   (c) Scarce Currency
   (d) Surplus Currency
3. **The State Election Commission conducts, controls and supervises Municipal elections under**
   (a) Article 240 (A)
   (b) Article 241 (B)
   (c) Article 243 (K)
   (d) Article 245 (D)
4. **Which committee was established on Criminal, Politician and Bureaucratic nexus ?**
   (a) Vohra Committee
   (b) Indrajit Gupta Committee
   (c) Tarkunde Committee
   (d) Santhanam Committee
5. **In which year was the Prevention of Terrorism Act (POTA) enacted ?**
   (a) 2000 (b) 2001
   (c) 2002 (d) 2003
6. **The first Atom bomb was dropped on Hiroshima on**
   (a) August 6, 1945
   (b) August 9, 1945
   (c) August 9, 1946
   (d) August 6, 1942
7. **'Indica' was authored by**
   (a) Kautilya (b) Megasthenes
   (c) Aryabhatta (d) Seleucus
8. **The world's largest island is**
   (a) Greenland
   (b) Madagascar
   (c) New Zealand
   (d) Sri Lanka
9. **The humidity of air depends on**
   (a) Temperature
   (b) Location
   (c) Weather
   (d) All of the above
10. **The 'Maasai' is a primitive tribe of**
    (a) Angola (b) Botswana
    (c) Nigeria (d) Tanzania
11. **Tropical rain forest is characterised by**
    (a) Absence of trees
    (b) Least productivity
    (c) Maximum biodiversity
    (d) Minimum biodiversity
12. **Enzymes are**
    (a) Proteins (b) Minerals
    (c) Oils (d) Fatty acids
13. **The largest cells in mammals blood are**
    (a) Erythrocytes
    (b) Monocytes
    (c) Basophils
    (d) Lymphocytes
14. **Who proposed Binomial Nomenclature?**
    (a) Linnaeus (b) John Ray
    (c) Huxley (d) Aristotle
15. **Who proposed Five Kingdom Classification ?**
    (a) R H . Whittaker
    (b) John Ray
    (c) Carolus Linnaeus
    (d) H.F. Copeland
16. **Which of the following have the same unit ?**
    (a) Work and power
    (b) Torque and moment of inertia
    (c) Work and torque
    (d) Torque and angular momentum
17. **Distances of stars are measured in**
    (a) Galactic unit
    (b) Stellar mile
    (c) Cosmic kilometre
    (d) Light year
18. **Loudness of sound depends on**
    (a) Frequency
    (b) Wavelength
    (c) Amplitude
    (d) Pitch
19. **What is the full form of ALU ?**
    (a) Alternative Logic Unit
    (b) Arithmetic Logic Unit
    (c) Arithmetic Least Unit
    (d) Arithmetic Local Unit
20. **Carborundum is another name of**
    (a) Silicon carbide
    (b) Silicon oxide
    (c) Calcium carbide
    (d) Calcium oxide
21. **Number of neutrons in an atom of hydrogen is**
    (a) One (b) Zero
    (c) Two (d) Three
22. **When the moon completely covers the sun, it is known as**

(a) the Antumbra
(b) the Umbra
(c) the Penumbra
(d) None of these

23. Who developed the model of atomic structure ?
(a) Bohr and Rutherford
(b) Volta
(c) Alfred Nobel
(d) Faraday

24. Which is the holy book of the Sikh religion ?
(a) Bhagwad Gita
(b) Baani
(c) Gurmukhi
(d) Guru Granth Sahib

25. Which of the following trophies is not awarded in cricket?
(a) Deodhar Trophy
(b) Ashes
(c) Ryder Cup
(d) Ranji Trophy

26. Which among the following comes under the tertiary sector of the Indian Economy?
(a) Cloth industry
(b) Transport of goods
(c) Dairy
(d) Sugar industry

27. ...... publishes Economic Survey in India.
(a) Government of India
(b) Ministry of Finance
(c) NITI Aayog
(d) Prime Minister of India

28. In which economic system does the government decide what goods are to be produced in accordance with the needs of society?
(a) Socialist (b) Mixed
(c) Capitalist (d) Traditional

29. 1 rupee note bears the signature of whom?
(a) Government of India
(b) Chief Justice of India
(c) Finance Secretary of India
(d) Prime Minister of India

30. Which five = year plan recognised human development as the core of all developmental efforts?
(a) First Five = Year Plan
(b) Second Five = Year Plan
(c) Eighth Five = Year Plan
(d) Ninth Five = Year Plan

Answers with Explanations

1. (c) The terms 'bull' and 'bear' describe upward and downward trends respectively of the stock market. A bear market refers to a decline in prices, usually for a period of a few months, in a single security or asset, group of securities or the securities market as a whole. A bull market is when prices are rising.

2. (b) Managed currency refers to currency whose exchange rate is not determined by the freemarket forces of demand and supply but instead by the government's intervention through the country's central bank. The majority of major world currencies are managed at least to some degree.

3. (c) According to Article 243 (K), the superintendence, direction and control of the preparation of electoral rolls for, and the conduct of, all elections to local bodies shall be vested in a State Election Commission consisting of a State Election Commissioner to be appointed by the Governor.

4. (a) The Vohra Committee (1993) studied the criminalization of politics and nexus among criminals, politicians and bureaucrats in India. It concluded that the existing criminal justice system is unable to deal with the activities of the politicians, police and the criminals as the provisions of law are emerging weak enough to fracture this nexus.

5. (c) The Prevention of Terrorism Act (POTA) was an Act passed by the Parliament of India in 2002, with the aim of strengthening anti-terrorism operations. It replaced the Prevention of Terrorism Ordinance (POTO) of 2001 and the Terrorist and Disruptive Activities (Prevention) Act (TADA) (1985-95).

6. (a) A uranium gun-type atomic bomb (Little Boy) was dropped on Hiroshima on August 6, 1945. It was followed by a plutonium implosion-type bomb (Fat Man) on the city of Nagasaki on August 9, 1945. The twin bombings led to Japan's surrender in the Second War.

7. (b) Indica was written by Megasthenes, a Greek historian, philosopher, and statesman during the Roman period. He stayed as a Greek envoy to the court of Chandragupta Maurya.

8. (a) Greenland is the world's largest island covering 2,175,597 square kilometers. New Guinea and Borneo come next. Greenland is located between the Arctic Ocean and the North Atlantic Ocean, northeast of Canada and northwest of Iceland.

9. (d) Humidity is the amount of water vapor in the air. Humidity depends on water vaporization, and condensation, which. In turn, mainly depends on temperature. Temperature, in turn, is affected by weather and location.

10. (d) The Maasai people of East Africa live in southern Kenya and northern Tanzania along the Great Rift Valley on semiarid and arid lands. Livestock such as cattle, goats and sheep are the primary source of income for the Maasai.

11. (c) Tropical rainforests exhibit high levels of biodiversity. Around 40% to 75% of all biotic species are indigenous to the rainforests. Rainforests are home to half of all the living animal and plant species on the planet. Two-thirds of all flowering plants can be found in rainforests.

12. (a) Enzymes are biological molecules (proteins) that act as catalysts and help complex reactions occur everywhere in life. They are in general globular proteins. They speed up reactions by providing an alternative reaction pathway of lower activation energy.

13. (b) Various components of blood are: Plasma, Erythrocytes (Red Blood Cells). Leucocytes (White Blood Cells) and Thrombocytes/Platelets. Monocytes, also known as macrophages, are the largest blood cells In most mammals, measuring 10-15 m in diameter. They are leucocytes. Their nuclei are kidney-shaped and cytoplasm is abundant.

14. (a) Binomial nomenclature is a formal system of naming species of living things by giving each a name composed of two parts, both of which use Latin grammatical forms. The formal introduction of this system of naming species is credited to Swedish natural scientist Carl Linnaeus, effectively beginning with his work 'Species Plantarum' in 1753.

15. (a) R.H Whittaker proposed the five kingdom classification in 1969. Those five kingdoms are: Monera, Protista, Mycota (Fungi). Metaphyta (Plantae) and Metazoa (Animalia). It is the most accepted system of modern classification as the different groups of animals are placed phylogenetically.

16. (c) The SI unit of work is the Newton-metre or joule (J). Newton meter is also the SI unit of torque (also called "moment" or "moment of force").

17. (d) Light year is a unit of length used informally to express astronomical distances. It is most often used when expressing distances to stars and other distances on a galactic scale. It is equal to just under 10 trillion kilometres.

18. (c) Loudness depends on the amplitude of the sound wave. The larger the amplitude the more energy the sound wave contains therefore the louder the sound. The pitch of a note depends on the frequency of the source of the sound.

19. (b) ALU stands for arithmetic logic unit which is the part of a computer processor (CPU) that carries out arithmetic and logic operations on the operands in computer instruction words. It is a fundamental building block of the central processing unit found in digital computers.

20. (a) Silicon carbide, also known as carborundum, is a compound of silicon and carbon with chemical formula SiC. It occurs in nature as the extremely rare mineral moissanite. Silicon carbide powder has been mass-produced since 1893 for use as an abrasive.

21. (b) Neutrons are the particles in an atom that have neutral charge. So, if an atom has equal numbers of electrons and protons, the charges cancel each other out and the atom has a neutral charge. Hydrogen (H) has 1 proton and 1 electron; it does not have any neutron in its nucleus.

22. (b) A solar eclipse occurs when the moon crosses the path between the sun and the earth. The darkest shadow (where the sun is completely covered) is called the umbra. The umbra is narrow at the distance of the Earth, and a total eclipse is observable only within the narrow strip of land or sea over which the umbra passes. The partial shadow is called the penumbra.

23. (a) In 1911, Ernest Rutherford used experimental evidence to show that an atom must contain a central nucleus. Niels Bohr further developed Rutherford's nuclear atom model. He used experimental evidence to support the idea that elections occupy particular orbits or shells around the nucleus of an atom.

24. (d) Guru Granth Sahib is the central religious text of Sikhism, considered by Sikhs to be the final, sovereign guru among the lineage of 11 Sikh Gurus of the religion. It is a voluminous text of 1430 pages, compiled and composed during the period of Sikh gurus from 1469 to 1708.

25. (c) The Ryder Cup is a biennial men's golf competition between teams from Europe and the United States. The competition is contested every two years with the venue alternating between courses in the USA and Europe. The Ryder Cup is named after the English businessman Samuel Ryder.

26. (b) The tertiary sector or service sector is the third of the three economic sectors of the three-sector theory. The tertiary sector of industry involves the provision of services to other businesses as well as final consumers. Services may involve the transport, distribution and sale of goods from a producer to a consumer as may happen in wholesaling and retailing, or may involve the provision of a service, such as in pest control or entertainment.

27. (b) The Department of Economic Affairs in the Finance Ministry of India publishes and presents the Economic Survey in the Parliament every year, just before the Union Budget. It is prepared under the guidance of the Chief Economic Adviser to Finance Ministry. It is the ministry's view on the annual economic development of the country.

28. (a) A socialist economic system is characterised by social ownership and democratic control of the means of production, which may mean autonomous cooperatives or direct public ownership; wherein production is carried out directly for use. Where markets are utilised for allocating inputs and capital goods among economic units, the designation market socialism is used. When planning is utilised, the economic system is designated a planned socialist economy.

29. (c) Under Section-22 of the Reserve Bank of India Act, RBI has sole right to issue currency notes of various denominations except one-rupee notes. The one-rupee note is issued by Ministry of Finance and it bears the signatures of Finance Secretary of India, while other notes bear the signature of the Governor the RBI.

30. (c) The National Development Council ratified the format of the Eighth Five-Year Plan. It was decided that the Eighth Five-Year Plan would commence on April 1, 1992. In this Five-Year Plan, the main objective of Eighth Five-Year Plan was creation of employment, check population growth, and overall human development as the core of all the development efforts, primary health facilities, drinking water and vaccination in all villages, growth and diversification of agricultural activities and strengthening the basic Infrastructure. Eight Plan was a plan for managing the transition from a centrally planned economy to market-led economy through indicative planning.

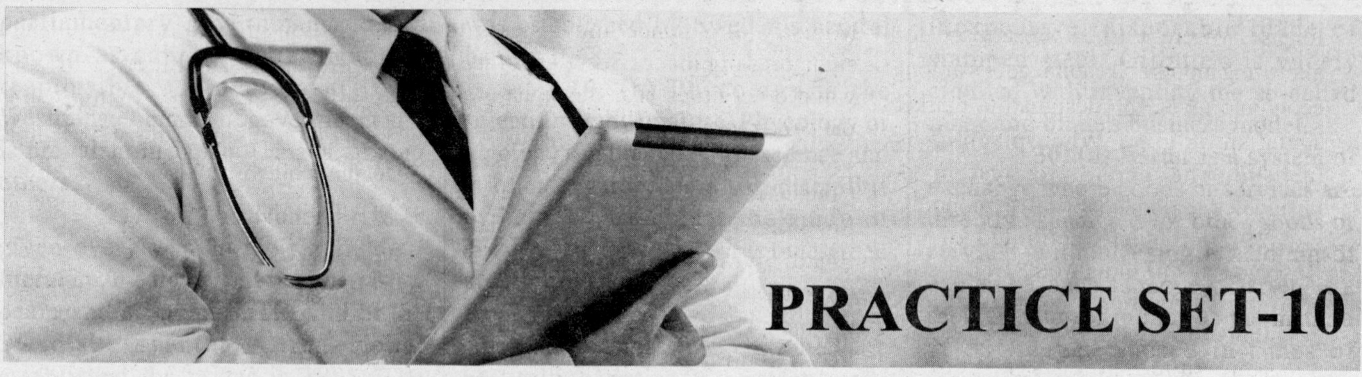

PRACTICE SET-10

1. Which one of the following is *not* a method for computing GNP?
(a) Income Approach
(b) Expenditure Approach
(c) Savings Approach
(d) Value Added Approach

2. Who said "Rama Rajya through Grama Rajya"?
(a) Mahatma Gandhi
(b) Vinoba Bhave
(c) Jayaprakash Narayan
(d) Jawaharlal Nehru

3. Where do we find the ideals of Indian democracy in the Constitution?
(a) The Preamble (b) Part III
(c) Part IV (d) Part I

4. Comptroller and Auditor General of India is appointed by the
(a) Prime Minister
(b) President
(c) Finance Minister
(d) Lok Sabha

5. Which Article of the Indian Constitution directs the State Governments to organise Village Panchayats?
(a) Article 32 (b) Article 37
(c) Article 40 (d) Article 51

6. The Attorney General of India has the right of audience in
(a) the Supreme Court
(b) any High Court
(c) any Sessions Court
(d) any Court of Law within India

7. The capital of the ancient Chola kingdom was
(a) Uraiyur
(b) Kaveripoompattinam
(c) Thanjavur
(d) Madurai

8. The Greater Himalayas is otherwise called
(a) Himadri
(b) Sahyadri
(c) Assam Himalayas
(d) Sivaliks

9. The cool temperate grasslands of South America are known as
(a) Pampas (b) Prairies
(c) Veldts (d) Savannah

10. Which of the biomes is called the "Bread Basket" of the world?
(a) Mid-latitude grasslands
(b) Taiga
(c) Mediterranean
(d) Tropical Savannah

11. Lactogenic hormone is secreted by
(a) mammary glands
(b) placenta
(c) ovary
(d) pituitary

12. An organism which can monitor air pollution is
(a) bacteria (b) lichen
(c) algae (d) fungi

13. In the human body, which of the following organs is responsible for water balance?
(a) Heart (b) Liver
(c) Kidneys (d) Lungs

14. Chlorophyll containing autotrophic thallophytes is called
(a) algae
(b) lichens
(c) fungi
(d) bryophytes

15. A white and smooth surface is
(a) good absorber and good reflector of heat
(b) bad absorber and good reflector of heat
(c) good absorber and bad reflector of heat
(d) bad absorber and bad reflector of heat

16. A computer programming language often used by children
(a) LOGO (b) PILOT
(c) BASIC (d) JAVA

17. A portable personal computer small enough to fit on your lap is called a
(a) note-book computer
(b) PDA
(c) mainframe computer
(d) workstation

18. Assembler is a program that translates the program from
(a) high level to assembly
(b) assembly to machine
(c) machine to low level
(d) low level to high level

19. Table sugar is which type of sugar?
(a) Fructose (b) Galactose
(c) Glucose (d) Sucrose

20. An alloy used in making heating elements for an electric heating device is
(a) solder (b) alloy Steel
(c) nichrome (d) german silver

21. The degree of dissociation of an electrolyte depends on
(a) dilution
(b) impurities
(c) atmospheric pressure
(d) method of dissolution

22. Chlorophyll contains
(a) iron
(b) magnesium
(c) cobalt
(d) zinc

23. Which one of the following days *is not* observed on a fixed date every year?
(a) World Environment Day
(b) International Women's Day
(c) International Friendship Day
(d) World Habitat Day

24. Which one of the following novels was a source of inspiration for the freedom fighters in India?
(a) Pariksha Guru
(b) Ananda Math
(c) Rangbhoomi
(d) Padmarag

25. Which one of the following monuments is the first inhabited World Heritage Monument?
(a) Agra Fort
(b) Red Fort
(c) Jaisalmer Fort
(d) Amber Fort

26. A system of rules that takes effect when a military authority takes control of the normal administration of justice is called
(a) Coup
(b) Strike
(c) Martial law
(d) Political prisoner

27. Who among the following is the most important political institution in a democratic country?
(a) President
(b) Parliament
(c) Prime Minister
(d) Cabinet Ministers

28. Which kind of decisions are usually based on careful calculation of gains and losses?
(a) Moral (b) Socialist
(c) Prudential (d) Ethnic

29. Emergency provisions in the Indian Constitution have been taken from the
(a) British Constitution
(b) Government of India Act, 1935
(c) Irish Constitution
(d) Japanese Constitution

30. Which of the following can be amended by special majority?
(a) Directive Principles of State Policy
(b) Rules of Procedure in the Parliament
(c) Admission of a new State
(d) Use of English language in the Parliament

Answers with Explanations

1. (a) Gross National Product (GNP) can be defined as an economic statistic which includes Gross Domestic Product plus any income earned by the residents from investments made overseas. Net factor income from abroad = Income earned in foreign countries by the residents of country – Income earned by non-residents in that country.

2. (a) Mahatma Gandhi advocated that Rama Rajya will not happen until Grama Rajya happens. He gave the ideology of 'Back to Villages'.

3. (a) The Preamble to the Constitution of India is 'Declaration of Independence' statement and a brief introductory that sets out the guiding principles and purpose of the document as well as Indian democracy. It describes the state as a "soverign democratic republic". The first part of the preamble "We the people of India" and, its last part "give to ourselves this Constitution" clearly indicate the democratic spirit.

4. (b) The Comptroller and Auditor-General of India is appointed by the President of India following a recommendation by the Prime Minister. On appointment, he/she has to make an oath or affirmation before the President of India.

5. (c) Article-40 directs the State to take steps to organise Village Panchayats and endow them with such powers and authority as may be necessary to enable them to function as units of self-government. It comes under Directive Principles of State Policy.

6. (d) The Attorney General has the right of audience in all Courts in India as well as the right to participate in the proceedings of the Parliament, though not to vote. He is the Indian government's chief legal advisor, and its primary lawyer in the Supreme Court of India.

7. (a) The Early Cholas of the pre-and post-Sangam period (3000 BCE-200 CE) were one of the three main kingdoms of the ancient Tamil country. Uraiyur, now Tiruchirappalli was the ancient capital of the Chola Dynasty.

8. (a) The Himalayas is divided into three major geographical entities, the Himadri (Greater Himalaya), Himanchal (Lesser Himalaya) and the Sivaliks (Outer Himalaya). These divisions extend almost uninterrupted throughout its length and are separated by major geological fault lines.

9. (a) The major temperate grasslands of the world include the Veldts of Africa, the Pampas of South America, the Steppes of Eurasia, and the plains of

North America. Pampas are mainly fertile South American lowlands found primarily in Argentina and extend into Uruguay.

10. (a) The mid-latitude grasslands are called the world's bread basket regions of grain and livestock production. They are found in the middle latitudes of South America, North America, Africa and Asia.

11. (d) Lactogenic hormone is gonadotrophic hormone which is secreted by the anterior pituitary. In females, it stimulates growth of the mammary glands and lactation after parturition.

12. (b) Lichens can be used as air pollution indicators, especially of the concentration of sulphur dioxide in the atmosphere. Air pollutants dissolved in rainwater, especially suphur dioxide, can damage lichens and prevent them from growing. This makes lichens natural indicators of air pollution.

13. (c) The kidneys maintain our body's water balance by controlling the water concentration of blood plasma. The kidneys also control salt levels and the excretion of urea.

14. (a) Algae are chlorophyll (green pigment) containing thallophytes. They prepare their own food and are, thus, autotrophic in their mode of nutrition.

15. (b) Shiny surfaces are poor absorbers of heat radiation and the best reflectors of heat radiation. Black surfaces are the best emitters and best absorbers of heat radiation.

16. (a) LOGO is a computer programming language used for functional programming, and is used for generating basic shapes using a turtle cursor. It was developed for children experimenting their first programming steps. It guides kids step by step with the basics of computer programming.

17. (a) Laptops are also sometimes called notebook computers or notebooks. They are portable personal computers with a clamshell form factor, suitable for mobile use. Other terms, such as ultrabooks or netbooks, refer to specific types of laptop/notebook.

18. (b) Assembler is a computer program which is used to translate a program written in assembly language into machine language. The translated program is called object program.

19. (d) Sucrose is the organic compound commonly known as table sugar and sometimes called saccharose. A white, odourless, crystalline powder with a sweet taste, it is best known for its role in food.

20. (c) Nichrome is a mixture of chromium and nickel. Nichrome wire is a great conductor of electricity. Nichrome is used to make heating coils and other types of elements in household appliances.

21. (a) The extent to which an electrolyte dissociates into ions is known as degree of dissociation or ionisation.

22. (b) Chlorophyll molecule contains a magnesium ion. Green plants are dependent on chlorophyll for photosynthesis, and magnesium is required for chlorophyll production.

23. (d) World Habitat Day is observed every year on the first Monday of October throughout the world. It was officially designated by the United Nations and first celebrated in 1986. World Environment Day: 5 June; International Women's Day: 8 March, International Friendship Day: 30 July.

24. (b) Ananda Math is a Bengali novel, written by Bankim Chandra Chatterjee and published in 1882. Set in the background of the Sannyasi Rebellion in the late 18th century, it became synonymous with the struggle for Indian independence from the British Empire. The famous song of India, Vande Mataram was first published in this novel.

25. (c) The Jaisalmer Fort in Rajasthan has become the first inhabited monument to have been declared a World Heritage Monument by UNESCO. At least, 450 families still reside in the fort complex.

26. (c) Martial law is the imposition of direct military control of normal civilian functions of the government, especially in response to a temporary emergency such as invasion or major disaster, or in an occupied territory. Martial law can be used by governments to enforce their rule over the public. All the administrative functions come under the control of the miltary and the Constitutional Rights of the people get violated everyday.

27. (c) The Prime Minister is the most important political institution in any democratic country. The Prime Minister is the leader of the country who represents the entire population of the country. Controlling the other economic variables, the main findings indicate that the political institutions fundamentally matter only for incipient democracies, and not for consolidated democracies. Political institutions demonstrate that consolidated democracies and political institutions are substituted for determining economic growth.

28. (c) The decisions which are taken usually based on careful calculation of gains and losses are called prudential. These types of decisions are contrasted with the decisions based purely on moral considerations. Prudential reasons stress that power-sharing will bring out better outcomes. Moral decisions are those decisions which are taken only on moral consideration. Moral reasons emphasise the very act of power-sharing as valuable.

29. (b) Many call the Indian Constitution a copy-paste work and a glaring example of plagiarism. Most parts of it have been copied from the Government of India Act, 1935. The emergency provision in the Constitution of India was borrowed from the Government of India Act, 1935. Some other provisions which are taken from this Act are Federal Scheme (also from the Constitution of Canada), Office of Governor, Judiciary and Public Service Commission.

30. (a) Any majority other than simple, absolute and effective majority, is called special majority. These include majority by two-third strength of the house (example impeachment of President under Article-61), majority by two-thirds of present and voting members (example: power of Parliament to legislate with respect to a matter in the State List in the national interest, under Article- 249); certain Constitution Amendment Bills etc. Absolute majority + majority of two-thirds present and voting (example: removal of Supreme Court Judge, CAG, and etc. and amendment in the Directive Principles of State Policy.